Cathedral of Healing

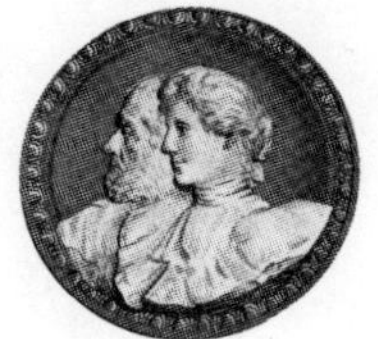

The Story of
Wesley Memorial Hospital
1888 to 1972

Vernon K. Brown

Northwestern Memorial Hospital
Chicago, Illinois

Library of Congress Cataloging in Publication Data

Brown, Vernon K.
   A cathedral of healing.

   Bibliography: p. 243
   Includes index.
   1. Wesley Memorial Hospital—History. I. Northwestern Memorial Hospital.
II. Title. (DNLM: 1. Hospitals, General—History—Chicago. WX 27 A13 B8c)
RA982.C452W473   362.1'1'0977311   81-4013
                                        AACR2
ISBN 0-9605996-1-4

Table of Contents

Preface

The joy of historical research is in building an established fact into a new concept that adds perspective and understanding to the present. It is known that Wesley Hospital was founded in 1888. This book records the events and conditions that brought about action, the people who initiated Wesley's origin and spurred its development, their wisdom, strength and faith which, all combined, set the institution on an unwavering course of service.

The Deaconess Nurse movement in Kaiserswerth, Germany, which had inspired Passavant Memorial Hospital's start in 1865, also made possible Wesley's beginning 23 years later. This discovery prompted the author to probe further and prepare a prologue chronicling hospital evolution leading directly to Wesley.

Research often reveals half-truths requiring re-examination to perceive the whole truth. For this reason, certain documents that previously may have been understood only in part, are printed in full herein for the reader's continued reference. Letters, which could have been condensed, are quoted so that the writer's context is preserved to clarify his meaning for the reader.

I am grateful to David L. Everhart, president of Northwestern Memorial Hospital, for the opportunity to write the Story of Chicago Wesley Memorial Hospital, the most challenging assignment of my thirty-year writing career. I began immediately after the history of Passavant was published in May, 1977. Although Passavant was 23 years older, Wesley was vastly more complicated with its earlier affiliation with Northwestern University Medical School and two mergers before the final union with Passavant, August, 1972, the end of their individual histories.

Descendants of early Wesley families, Dr. David Newton Danforth, Wesley M. Dixon, and Edward F. Swift III showed sustained interest in helping to unravel some of the difficult historical threads and in reading the complete manuscript. It was gratifying to receive letters approving the manuscript from J. Deering Danielson and Brooks McCormick, nephews of James Deering, Wesley's major benefactor. Dr. Leslie B. Arey, emeritus professor of anatomy at Northwestern and author of the medical school history made helpful suggestions after reviewing the prologue and chapters germane to the medical school. Kenath Hartman, executive vice-president, provided important information through interviews and the loan of pertinent papers obtained during his tenure as chief executive officer.

Many persons on the hospital staff gave valuable assistance. Curt Thompson, public relations director, made available the graphic arts facilities employed by his department. Judi Rice, associate director of public relations and editorial assistant, served as liaison officer with the designer and printer. Ira Berlin, hospital archivist, gathered resource material including documents, minutes, letters, Wesley publications, newspaper/magazine articles, books, and photos. Evelyn Geis, who was indexer for the Passavant book, served in the same capacity for Wesley.

My heartfelt appreciation goes to my husband, Madison B. Brown, M.D., for his infinite patience in reading each chapter with special attention to medical and administrative accuracy. The availability of his personal medical library and that of his alma mater, the University of Vermont Medical School, provided the sources for the prologue.

Vernon Kimball Brown

Prologue
Hospitals Through the Ages:
The Interrelation of Medical Science,
Nursing and Facilities

Each hospital possesses a distinct character molded by its own traditions and the environment of its origin. Yet the hospital also follows the mainstream of civilization, reflecting the culture and the knowledge of its time. In the past the current seemed to move according to prevailing emotions. Compassion, piety and love usually accompanied the quest for knowledge, improved living standards, concern for one another and advances in health care and hospitals. Fear, prejudice and repression were associated with pestilence, famine and other catastrophes together with retrogression of medical care and hospitals.

Throughout history, the three ingredients essential to an effective and responsible hospital have been medical science, compassionate nursing care and efficient facilities. These three factors are interdependent; weakness in any one of the triad cripples the whole institution.

A hospital's history begins long before the lives of its founders and even those of their predecessors. It evolves from the start of civilization which itself is antedated first by individual self-interest, then concern for the family and finally for the community.

Civic awareness and religious fervor led men and women to build retreats for the sick thousands of years ago. War, too, played a significant part in the development of care for the disabled. A limestone pillar dating back to the Sumerians (2920 B.C.) portrays a gathering of the wounded, presumably for treatment, among carvings of military procedures.

Hindu literature reveals that Buddha, in about 600 B.C., appointed a physician for every ten villages and built hospitals for the disabled. Physicians were required to bathe daily, keep hair and nails short, wear white garments and respect the confidence of their patients.[1] Facilities were crude but physicians applied their utmost skills, attendants were instructed to give gentle care and the buildings met the standards of the era. They had the necessary elements of a hospital and undoubtedly pain was alleviated and lives saved.

GREEK AND ROMAN HOSPITALS

Temples of the pagan gods were used as refuge for the sick in early Greek and Roman settlements where medical practice was imbued with mysticism and superstition. Snakes were sacred and thought to have magical powers which physicians called upon in treatment. They are said to have used the tongues of serpents in cleansing ulcers. From such origins possibly came the *caduces*, formed by two snakes entwined around a staff, symbol of the physician today.

Ruins have been found of a temple at Titanus built around 1134 B.C., dedicated to Aesculapius, Greek god of Medicine, and used to succor the sick. Other ruins exist of a Greek temple built several centuries later in the Hieron or sacred grove at Episaurus. Here hot and cold baths were given and salt, honey and water from a sacred spring were prescribed. An immense gymnasium was used by thousands of persons for gymnasiotherapy, forerunner of physical therapy in hospitals today. The Greeks were first with medical records, as may be seen on the columns of the temple at Epidaurus, where the names of patients with brief case histories and results are engraved.

Throughout the Greek islands, Aesculapia with therapeutic programs similar to those of Epidaurus were built. One of the most popular was the

---

[1]*Fielding H. Garrison, Introduction to the History of Medicine*

temple at Kos, the town where Hippocrates, known today as the "father of medicine," was born in 460 B.C.

Hippocrates renounced the medical myths of Aesculapius, insisting that his followers see and *reason* about what they saw for the sole purpose of curing the sick. His ethics were exalted and out of them evolved the "Hippocratic Oath."[1] He died at the age of 90 or more at Larissa in Thessaly. His work continued through Celsus, Antyllus and Galen, the last of the great Greek doctors. Galen was born at Pergamus in 130 A.D. He studied, traveled and began practice in Rome. Galen wrote 78 books and 14 essays on anatomy, physiology, pathology and therapeutics before he died at about 80 years of age. No physician surpassed Galen for a thousand years and his writings were considered the "perfection of medicine."

The Aesculapia continued to spread throughout the Roman empire where priest-physicians in the temples treated and instructed medical students. Galen wrote of the "tabernae medicae" where only the ambulatory sick were treated, probably the original outpatient clinic. The Romans had another custom that lasted: endowing hospitals. This was revealed when a tablet inscribed in recognition of a donor's generosity, dated at the time of Trajan (circa 100 A.D.), was found near Piacenza. During that era, hospitals and patient care were more like today's medical institutions than they would be again for fifteen centuries.

EARLY RELIGIOUS HOSPITALS

Research shows that many ancient hospitals were temples dedicated to the gods of medicine, with patient care accompanied by mystical pagan rites. With the advent of Christianity and its teachings of love and pity, the desire to help those less fortunate was intensified and Christian hospitals began to replace those in the temples of Greece and Italy. Patients were accommodated in buildings outside the church itself and many followers of the teachings of Jesus devoted themselves entirely to the care of the sick.

In 335 A.D., Constantine decreed that the Aesculapia be closed and replaced by Christian hospitals. Rulers of the fourth and fifth centuries erected numerous such edifices. The greatest of these was Justinian's Hospital of St. Basil at Caesarea erected in 369 A.D., a medical center for the sick and aged. Women took an active part in early Christian hospitals.

[1] *Grove Wilson, Great Men of Science*

In Constantinople, two affluent women who were deaconesses[1] in the church, devoted their time to nursing the sick; in Rome a prominent matron, Fabiola, endowed a public hospital in 390 A.D. Nearly 2000 years later, knowledge of the deaconesses in the early church had an impact on the founding of Wesley Hospital (see page 15) and Passavant Memorial Hospital in Chicago.

Christian hospitals continued to be erected until, by 500 A.D., almost every large town in the Roman empire had such an institution. Tragically, the medical expertise of Hippocrates and Galen was discarded because it was of pagan origin. But nursing, inspired by Christianity, was gentle and compassionate. In this period, nursing and facilities excelled but the other necessary factor, medical science, declined and hospitals retrogressed.

Little is known about care of the sick in Europe during the next six centuries, except in the hospitals previously mentioned and two notable ones in France: the Hotel Dieu of Lyons, founded in 542 A.D., and the Hotel Dieu of Paris, founded in 660 A.D. Although destroyed and rebuilt at different locations several times, the Paris institution has given continued service since its opening. In addition to care for the sick, these French hospitals or hotels, as they were called, offered shelter to travelers.

The etymology of the three words, "hospital," "hotel," and "hostel" reveals that all are from the same Latin source. Now carrying different meanings, all were once synonymous.[2]

The Mohammedans rivaled the Christians in providing health care for their people. A Jewish traveler in Baghdad around 1160 reported that he found sixty dispensaries and infirmaries in the city alone. Under

---

[1]*"Deaconess" is the English translation from the Greek word, diakonos, meaning one who gives prompt and helpful service. In the New Testament the first "deaconess" ("diakonos" or "diakonon") mentioned is Phoebe who is given a special introduction by the apostle Paul in his letter to the Romans: "I commend to you our sister Phoebe, a deaconess of the church at Cenchreae, that you may receive her in the Lord as befits the saints, and help her in whatever she may require from you, for she has been a helper of many and of myself as well." Romans 16.1-2, Revised Standard Version, 1946, Holy Bible. Some earlier versions interpret "diakonos" as "servant".*

[2]*The words "hospital" and "hotel" are derived from the Latin "hospitalis" (adjective) and "hospes" (noun) meaning host or guest. The French "hospice" came from the Latin "hospitium," a place in which a guest was received. "Hospitalis" and "hospitale" became "hospital" and "hospitalia." The English word "hospital" comes from the old French "Hospitale" as do "hostel" and "hotel" all originally from the Latin.*

Mohammedan control, the cities of Cairo, Damascus, Cordova and others all provided the highest quality of medical care then known.

The Arabians were expert chemists and developed a large number of drugs. They studied the possibilities of anesthesia by inhalation and they had asylums for the mentally ill a thousand years before they appeared in Europe.

MEDIEVAL HOSPITALS

Renewed religious zeal in the tenth century was apparent in the establishment of hospitals which were more ecclesiastical than medical. The church forbade opening the human body and sought to cure the ill through faith and love without regard for scientific knowledge and skill. Many religious orders opened hospitals next to monasteries which offered shelter and food to travelers along with care of the sick.

When the Crusades began around 1096, disease and pestilence were rampant. Hospitals were constructed along well traveled roads to provide care for exhausted and sick crusaders. The Hospitallers of the Order of St. John built a hospital in the Holy Land in 1099 which accommodated 2000 patients. Knights of the Order cared for patients personally, often denying themselves to give food and medications to the sick.

Hospitals were built in nearly every country in Europe during the 12th and 13th centuries. This increased activity was inspired by Pope Innocent III who, in 1198, urged citizens of important cities to subscribe to Hospitals of the Holy Spirit. He set the precedent by building a model hospital in Rome, the Santo Spirito, in 1204 which survived until 1922 when it was destroyed by fire. In Germany alone, 155 towns established Hospitals of the Holy Spirit during the Middle Ages. The papacy assisted them by levying a tax on one commercial item in each town for funds for the local hospital.

Most medieval city hospitals, like cathedrals, were colorfully decorated with tapestries and stained glass windows which gave almost no light. Patients occupied beds lining each side of drafty halls with only the cupola in the ceiling for ventilation. Some of the better hospitals of the Middle Ages were built in the form of a cross and had patient accommodations arranged in the ward plan.

Victims of leprosy, which had spread throughout Europe, were isolated in crude structures on the outskirts of towns. They were nursed by members of the Order of St. Lazar who controlled and nearly eradicated leprosy through isolation.

Three great London hospitals built during the middle ages were St. Bartholomew's (1137), St. Thomas (1206), and St. Mary of Bethlehem (1247). St. Mary of Bethlehem, the first English hospital to be used exclusively for the mentally ill, was shortened to Beddelem and later to Bedlem, adding a new word to the English language. St. Bartholomew's was founded by Rahere, said to have been the court jester of King Henry I. St. Thomas was founded by a woman with wealth she accumulated while operating a ferry across the Thames.

The Dark Age of Patient Care

In the late medieval period the church, which had fostered the founding of nearly all hospitals and had encouraged treating patients with kindness and love, also contributed to the deterioration of medical care.

In this dark age following the crusades, only monks and clergymen were educated, hence they usually were the physicians. A church edict of 1163 forbade the clergy to perform operations which required bloodshed. Later decrees limiting clergymen even further rendered them ineffective in the practice of medicine. Thus, those qualified to use the knowledge of Hippocrates and Galen were replaced by men equipped solely to apply the leech, a "treatment" they used continually.

Nursing care degenerated and many religious orders, on becoming wealthy, forgot their precepts of love and pity to emulate self-serving clerics. In hospitals, several patients were crowded into one bed without regard to type or seriousness of illness. A sick woman and child might be placed in bed with a man, terminally ill of a contagious disease, and awaken to find a corpse beside them.

During the decline of medicine, monks copied by hand the writings of Hippocrates and his followers. Thus the medical teachings of the ancient physicians were preserved in monasteries during the dark ages.

Quest for Knowledge Revives in Europe

A rebirth of learning came to Western Europe at the end of the fourteenth century. Medieval hospitals began to adopt the new techniques developed by Renaissance physicians.[1] Such barbaric instruments as the cautery iron were abolished, anatomy became a recognized study and old Greek medical writings were printed. Leonardo da Vinci illustrated the human body in anatomical drawings often used today to symbolize the medical field.

The revival in medical education began in Italy where students were permitted to walk the hospital wards for clinical observation under the supervision of experienced surgeons.[2] French and English hospitals soon adopted this teaching practice. Documents of a civil hospital in Padua (1569), which became Europe's most progressive medical school of the sixteenth century, show enlightened regulations relating to medical staff duties. They stated: "There shall be a doctor of physic upon whom rests the duty of visiting all the poor patients in the building, females as well as males; a doctor of surgery whose duty it is to apply ointments to all the poor people in the hospital who have wounds of any kind ..."

In the early sixteenth century, the small number of physicians permitted to do all types of surgical procedures had been educated in universities and were called "long robe surgeons."[3] In 1506 a group of them banded together and formed the Royal College of Surgeons of Edinburgh. Thomas Linacre, personal physician to King Henry VIII, organized English physicians in 1528 to form the Royal College of Physicians of England. Thus began professional societies which today assist in elevating standards and disseminating knowledge in the health field.

ENGLISH HOSPITALS ORDERED CLOSED

Hospitals began to retrogress in 1534. After King Henry was excommunicated for divorcing Catherine of Aragon, his first wife, the king claimed authority over the Catholic Church in England and the country emerged as Protestant. Because of their previous association with the Catholic Church, hospitals fell into disfavor with the crown and Henry ordered them used for secular purposes or destroyed.

Patients were turned out into the street and conditions became so deplorable that citizens pledged support and petitioned the king to return

[1]*Malcolm T. MacEachern, History of Hospitals*
[2]*Ibid*
[3]*Ibid*

at least one building for care of the most critically ill. Henry consented and ordered St. Bartholomew's, England's first great hospital, restored in 1544. He even appointed his personal surgeon, Thomas Vicary, as resident medical governor. Two other historic London hospitals, St. Thomas and St. Mary of Bethlehem, survived, but in other parts of England there were no general hospitals until 1710.

A contribution, unique for the times, was made to nursing when the order, Daughters of Charity of St. Vincent de Paul, was founded in France in 1634. It began at the Hotel Dieu in Paris where nuns trained a group of village girls in nursing care. The order grew and spread to America where it continues to serve today.

In England, poverty delayed construction of hospitals but a few were built and supported jointly by parishes. One of these was St. Peter's Hospital of Bristol, which was built early in the eighteenth century and served continually until November, 1940, when it was destroyed by war.

The Royal College of Physicians established a dispensary in about 1710 where advice was given free and medicine sold to the needy at cost. Other free medical dispensaries were established after 1745 by John Wesley,[1] the physician and theologian who traveled throughout the English countryside performing his evangelistic work.

A few English Hospitals were opened, Guy's Hospital in London (1725), Middlesex Hospital (1745), and Manchester Hospital (1753). England, however, having created the United Kingdom in 1707 by uniting with Scotland and Wales, appeared more interested in territorial acquisitions than in the people's health.

Although education, the arts, mechanical inventions and general culture had progressed rapidly during the 18th century and the first half of the 19th century, the care of patients in hospitals declined to its lowest ebb. The large, cold wards were seldom cleaned, the air was foul and patients were treated roughly and without consideration. The Renaissance did not come to hospitals until after 1850.

On the North American Continent

The Spanish built a hospital at Mexico City in 1524, the first health facility

---

[1]*Founder of the Methodist faith for whom several hospitals, including Wesley Hospital in Chicago, were named.*

on the North American Continent. The building stands today as a credit to the conquerors for attention to the ill and for architectural ability. In Canada, the first hospital, the Hotel Dieu du Precieux Sang, was founded in Quebec by the Duchess d'Aguilon in 1639. Five years later, a French noblewoman, Jeanne Mance, who had dedicated her life to religious work on the American frontier, established a hospital built of logs on the island of Montreal, now the city. Jeanne Mance also founded the Order of Sisters of St. Joseph, said to be the first group of nurses in North America.

In United States territory, the first hospital recorded was on Manhattan Island, established for sick and injured soldiers in 1663, a hundred years before the era of the American Revolution. Several colonial towns had almshouses, but usually the sick were nursed in their homes and given primitive medical care by families and neighbors.

The Pennsylvania Hospital, first incorporated hospital in America, was founded by Dr. Thomas Bond to provide facilities for Philadelphia physicians to treat charity patients. King George II granted a charter to Benjamin Franklin in 1751. Franklin also helped design the building and served as president of the hospital from its opening in 1755 until 1757.

New York City, with a population of 300,000, had no hospital in 1771 when Dr. John Jones and a group of citizens formed the Society of the New York Hospital. They were granted a charter for a model hospital with only eight beds to a ward, good ventilation and the best hospital facilities known at the time. English citizens assisted by subscribing to the building fund. Fire damaged the interior when the hospital was nearly completed, but it was rebuilt and completed in 1776. During the Revolutionary War British troops used the new structure as a military hospital and barrack for lodging soldiers.

In the southern states, South Carolina was among the first to provide hospital care. In 1829 a Charleston citizen, Colonel Thomas Roper, bequeathed funds for a community hospital "to provide for the permanent reception or occasional relief of all such sick, maimed, and diseased paupers as need surgical or medical aid...without regard to complexion, religion, or nation."[1] Roper Hospital continues today to meet the terms of the bequest.

[1]*Audio-visual presentation, opening plenary session, American Hospital Association, 76th annual convention, Atlanta*

Return To Ignorance and Pain

Hospitals had been built in most cities and the knowledge of centuries was available, yet medical error and prejudice turned the time between 1750 and 1850 into a dark and painful century for the sick. Surgeons knew anatomy well enough to perform many operations, but the mortality rate was often 90 and even 100 percent.

While ancient physicians had kept wounds clean, even using wine as an antiseptic, and had worn white garments and stressed hygiene, early 19th century surgeons believed that suppuration (the formation of pus) was beneficial. They called it "laudable pus" and even encouraged it. Hospital wards were so offensive with the stench of discharging wounds that nurses were said to use snuff to tolerate conditions. The same sheets served several patients and surgeons wore their operating coats for months without having them laundered. Hemorrhage, infection, gangrene and untold pain were the usual lot of the surgical patient.

Nursing was on an even lower level than medicine and surgery. The religious attendants of the previous century who nursed with love and pity had been replaced with lay people, often criminals, who exploited and mistreated the patients. The hospitals' administrators, accustomed to the free devoted service of sisters and deaconesses of the church, demanded unreasonably hard work and long hours of the lay people. This created a predicament that would not be resolved for several generations.

The Renaissance of Nursing

The light first dawned on nursing in Germany at the village of Kaiserswerth on the Rhine. There Theodore Fliedner, pastor of a small Protestant congregation, brought the primitive Order of Deaconesses again into existence after a thousand years of oblivion.

While on a tour of England, the Reverend Fliedner met Elizabeth Fry, whose work in relieving punitive conditions in British prisons was gaining recognition. He returned home in 1833 and found that convicts in German prisons were treated similarly. Pity, especially for the mistreated women prisoners, inspired Fliedner and his wife to open their home to discharged women convicts. From this simple beginning evolved a great system of hospitals, schools and orphanages which spread throughout Europe, Asia Minor, Northern Africa and Europe.

Soon the number of women seeking refuge after prison abuse exceeded the capacity of the modest Fliedner home. A small group called the Rhenish Westphalian Society was formed to assist the project. The society purchased a large nearby house which Fliedner opened as a hospital in 1836. The first young women assistants were drawn from the pastor's congregation. They became Deaconess Nurses, following the selfless compassionate precepts of the early Christian church. The Reverend Fliedner stressed that his workers were to be true "ministrae" or female ministers in charge. Some of the deaconess nurses developed into efficient hospital administrators and others dedicated themselves to bedside care.

The urgent need for nurses throughout Europe sent many hospital representatives to Kaiserswerth to observe the work of the devoted deaconesses and, when possible, to engage their services to set up similar systems in other cities. King Frederick William IV of Prussia and his wife became patrons of the unique institution and established a similar one in Berlin. Generous gifts enabled Fliedner's institution to increase its service.

Among the most interested visitors from abroad was a young Lutheran pastor, William Alfred Passavant from Pittsburgh, Pennsylvania, who had been attending an Evangelical Alliance in London. When he visited Kaiserswerth he immediately saw the possibilities of an American counterpart and he persuaded the Reverend Fliedner to assist. In 1849 Fliedner and four deaconess nurses arrived in Pittsburgh and helped Passavant open a Deaconess Hospital, the first in America under Protestant sponsorship, to be followed by hospitals in Milwaukee, Chicago, and Jacksonville, Illinois. The Deaconess Hospital established in Chicago in 1865 became Passavant Memorial Hospital following the founder's death June 3, 1894.[1]

In 1846 while the Reverend Passavant was marveling at Fliedner's achievements, another young person, Florence Nightingale of England, was beginning a nursing career at Kaiserswerth. Upon completion she applied her training, along with her own ideas, in London hospitals where she gained a reputation for organizational efficiency. In 1854 the English government appointed her to organize nursing in the military hospital in the Crimea. Miss Nightingale and a small group she had selected to assist her, found wounded British soldiers lying on vermin-infested straw beds

_____

[1] *This hospital merged with Chicago Wesley Memorial Hospital in 1972.*

covered with dirty canvas sheets. The proficient young nurse and her staff organized diet kitchens, a laundry, supplies, and brought order and cleanliness to the hospital within two weeks. As a result, the death rate was said to have been reduced from forty percent to two percent. In 1860 when the remarkable nurse returned to London she established the Nightingale School for Nursing at St. Thomas Hospital. In 1863, the school graduated a class of fifteen nurses who are said to have become the pioneer heads of schools of nursing throughout Europe.

The deaconess movement was adopted by women in other Protestant denominations including the Baptist, Congregational, Lutheran, Methodist and Presbyterian. Except for the Lutheran deaconesses recruited through Dr. Passavant, the young women in America were not specifically trained to nurse the sick; their major service was with orphans, the aged and the poor. The first formal instruction for these women was provided by the Chicago Training School for City, Home and Foreign Missions, established in 1885 under the auspices of the Methodist Episcopal Church of America. The school was started through the efforts of Lucy Rider Meyer and her husband, the Reverend Josiah Shelley Meyer, through whom forty charitable institutions were founded during their lifetimes. The need for missionaries to be trained as nurses led the Meyers to establish the Chicago Deaconess Home from which developed the Wesley Hospital in 1888.[1]

New Life for Hospitals

Two discoveries of the mid-19th century transformed hospitals from places synonymous with pain, infection and death into centers where medical science, skilled physicians and trained nurses save lives and preserve health. These crucial discoveries were *anesthesia* and the principles of *antisepsis*, (the destruction of the microorganisms that cause disease) and *asepsis* (the state of being free of those organisms).

The first published account of a successful operation on a patient under anesthesia occurred in Massachusetts General Hospital at Boston on October 16, 1846. Dr. William Thomas Green Morton, 1819-1868, a dentist and Harvard medical student, administered sulfuric ether to a 20-year-old printer with a tumor on the left side of his jaw. A full attendance of

---

[1]*Thus both Wesley Hospital and Passavant Memorial Hospital evolved from the same source of enlightened patient care—The Deaconess Hospital in Kaiserswerth on the Rhine.*

Harvard medical students observed Dr. John Collins Warren perform the usually extremely painful removal of the tumor. After surgery, the patient said he had felt no discomfort at all. The following year in England, Sir James Simpson used chloroform as an anesthetic for an obstetrical patient.

The discovery of the principles of antisepsis and asepsis occurred in the same year, 1847, at the Vienna Lying-In Hospital.[1] Dr. Ignaz Philipp Semmelweis observed that the frightening percentage of deaths from puerperal fever after childbirth was caused by medical students who transmitted infection from the dissecting room by going directly to examine obstetrical patients.[2] As colleagues ridiculed him, Semmelweis used his own antiseptic technique (washing hands in chlorine water before entering the maternity ward) and saw the mortality rate of his obstetrical patients drop to about one-ninth of what it had been. About 30 years later, Louis Pasteur in France provided an explanation for the success of Semmelweis. In 1879, Pasteur proved that bacteria were produced by reproduction and not by "spontaneous generation" as was then believed.

Joseph Lister worked vigorously on the problem at the Royal Infirmary at Glasgow. He concluded that suppuration, or pus formation, was caused by putrefaction or decomposition, which was set up by exposure of the wound to air, or by other contamination. A simple fracture, when skin was not broken, did not suppurate; when the skin was broken, it did. Lister used crude carbolic acid as a disinfectant and heat to sterilize instruments, bringing about dramatic decreases in postoperative fatalities.

Lister devoted his later life to lectures and demonstrations at Glasgow and London, trying to convince the medical world that suppuration was dangerous and "laudable pus" did not exist.[3] The two discoveries, anesthesia, which originated in America, and the principles of asepsis, British in origin, were slowly accepted, perfected, and used as stepping stones toward the achievements that take place in operating rooms today.

Health care was further advanced in 1847 when the American Medical Association (AMA) was formed partly through the efforts of Dr. Nathan Smith Davis, national exponent of medical education reform. At a meeting of the New York State Medical Society in 1846, Dr. Davis proposed that a

[1]*David Newton Danforth, "Historical Highlights," Textbook of Obstetrics and Gynecology*
[2]*Ibid*

[3]*A.G.L. Ives, British Hospitals*

committee be named to recommend a national medical association. The result was the founding of AMA, a forward step toward elevating standards in medical practice, education and hospitals. Dr. Davis was elected AMA president in 1864 and became editor of its journal in 1883.

Among the numerous accomplishments of Dr. Nathan Smith Davis, according to his friend and confrère, Dr. Isaac N. Danforth, none was more far-reaching than the radically different curriculum which he helped institute at the Chicago Medical College, which later became the Northwestern University Medical School. A leading pioneer in pathology, Dr. Danforth was author of the biography of Dr. Davis and the founder of Wesley Hospital in Chicago.

Danforth wrote about the significance of the new curriculum to the medical world in his book *The Life of Nathan Smith Davis, M.D., 1817-1904:*

> "The 9th of October, 1859, must always be regarded as an important epoch in the history of American medicine, and in the history of Chicago. On that day in a rather obscure city in the then remote and little known west . . . there was inauguarated a movement that was an acute and radical departure from the traditional and venerable methods of teaching . . ."

Dr. Danforth evaluated the results 33 years later:

> "One by one, slowly, many times doubtfully, many more times unwillingly, the medical schools of our country came to adopt the tripod which was the foundation of Dr. Davis' scheme, namely, the enforcement of a standard of preliminary education; the adoption of longer annual courses of college and clinical instruction, and the graded curriculum by which a definite number of branches are assigned to each year . . ."

The mainstream of health care was changing its course because physicians of the future were increasing their knowledge. Existing hospitals and those to come would follow in the current, cleansed in the light of science and truth—concepts of Drs. Davis and Danforth, with their colleagues.

These concepts were the roots of Chicago Wesley Memorial Hospital, roots that would produce a heritage of brilliant advances, some periods of regression, and finally a blend of professional skills and community support that mark hospitals of today.

Men of Vision in A New Metropolis

Chapter 1

Wesley Hospital, like other efficient and valuable enterprises, is largely the product of one man's brains and that man is Isaac Newton Danforth, M.D." This emphatic statement appeared under the title, "Wesley Hospital Reminiscences - not entirely adapted for a Conference Address," by Marcus P. Hatfield, M.D., dated October 6, 1899. The paper, which stressed the part religion played in Wesley's origin, continued, "A tripod consisting of Methodist money, knowledge and piety should have constituted a support strong enough to have carried even a weightier enterprise, but which of these supports grew uncertain during the next ten years, let the history of this hospital tell."

DR. DANFORTH: COMMENTS ON PAST AND FUTURE
Ten years later, Dr. Danforth was asked to prepare an account of the "vicissitudes of Wesley's callow days and of its development into a strong and successful institution." Agreeing in part with his early colleague, Dr. Danforth began, "It is urged that I write this since I was, to a considerable degree, the most active instrument in Wesley's formation. I probably know more about its early history than anyone else now living and should not delay placing on record my knowledge of the causes and events which led to the beginning of Wesley as an institution de facto..."

Dr. Danforth stated that his only objection to the task was the necessity of injecting himself into the report more than he found agreeable. "But I have concluded to waive that objection," he added, "with the comment that if anyone accuses me of egotism, I must admit that the 'prima facie' evidence is against me, and leave my justification to the future." The "future" has revealed that not only was Dr. Danforth the guiding force and inspiration of Wesley Hospital's founding, but a foremost pioneer in the science of pathology, an authority on renal disease and a prominent clinician and author.

Isaac Newton Danforth was born in Barnard, Vermont, in 1835 and was graduated from Dartmouth Medical School in Hanover, New Hampshire, in 1862. He interrupted his schooling in 1861 to volunteer in the Union Army, but was rejected as being "too short, underweight, coughing, and probably consumptive." He set up a successful practice in Greenfield, New Hampshire, but poor practice standards and the professional inertia of contemporaries prompted him to seek a larger area with brighter horizons. In preparation, he did postgraduate work at the University of Pennsylvania.

Danforth came from a long line of physicians. Of the nine ancestors who were physicians, one, Dr. Samuel Danforth, was physician to the American Revolution patriot, Paul Revere, whom he cared for in Revere's later years until his death in 1818 at the age of 83.

AHEAD OF HIS TIME

Dr. Danforth arrived in Chicago in 1866 and was said to be the city's first physician to own a microscope adequate by today's standards. He was appointed pathologist at St. Luke's Hospital in 1870 and two years later became an attending physician, a position he retained until his resignation in 1895. He became proficient in histology and in microscopic pathology and was, in 1877, appointed the first pathologist of the Cook County Hospital. He initiated an important advance in medical education by demonstrating postmortem examinations to medical students. Dr. Danforth resigned the Cook County post to create a vacancy for Dr. Christian Fenger[1] who had more than proved his qualifications to continue and expand Dr. Danforth's innovations.

---

[1]*Vernon K. Brown, The Story of Passavant Memorial Hospital, pages 38-39*

Dr. Danforth was a lecturer at Rush Medical Center where students considered him "fluent, often witty, and always bright and interesting." In 1881 he was recalled to Dartmouth to receive an honorary degree of Master of Arts and, in the same year, became a founding member and later president of the Chicago Pathological Society. From 1882 to 1897 he was professor of clinical medicine in the Chicago Medical College (later Northwestern University Medical School) and was dean of the faculty and professor of internal medicine of the Woman's Medical School of Northwestern.

In 1869 Dr. Isaac Danforth was married to Miss Elizabeth Skelton, a school teacher from England. A cherished memento of her teaching days was a note from Mary Todd Lincoln requesting that Tad (Thomas, fourth son of Mary Todd and Abraham Lincoln) be excused for absence from school because of illness. The Isaac Danforths had two children: a daughter, Esther, and a son, William Clark Danforth, who became a physician as did his son, David Newton Danforth.

ACCEPTS SURGICAL DISCOVERIES

Dr. Danforth was among the first of Chicago's physicians to accept the theories of aseptic (cleanliness, not only of instruments and surgeons' hands, but also of operating room and air) and antiseptic (destruction of microorganisms with disinfectants) surgical techniques.

Dr. Danforth had been convinced in 1872 through demonstrations and successful self-inoculations with catarrh (discharge from mucous membrane) that the germ hypothesis of the French bacteriologist, Louis Pasteur, went far to explain the nature of disease.[1] This had led the English physician, Joseph Lister, to perceive that the role of bacteria in wound pus might be causative rather than incidental. This hypothesis caused Lister to develop antiseptic surgery, first by using a layer of carbolic putty and then a carbolic spray to protect fresh wounds from invasion by microorganisms. In accepting the germ hypotheses of Pasteur and Lister, Dr. Danforth admitted that the "idea of such multitudes of parasitic tenants seem, at first sight, revolting and unendurable."[2] Unfortunately, the majority of physicians in Chicago did not concur for nearly a decade.

[1] *Thomas Neville Bonner, Medicine in Chicago 1850-1950, page 34*
[2] *Ibid*

New Techniques become Routine

As pathologist at Cook County Hospital in 1878, Dr. Danforth made antisepsis and asepsis part of the routine. His successor, Christian Fenger,[1] who became a world-famed surgeon-pathologist, continued these regulatory techniques, teaching that "cleanliness is the best and most efficient antiseptic."

By 1890, instruments were disinfected and gloves used in the operating rooms of most Chicago hospitals. Dr. Fenger was the first surgeon to use the rubber gloves in Chicago after discarding silk and cotton as unsuitable.

It was generally accepted that specific bacteria were responsible for specific diseases. This inspired a microbe hunt which would reveal the germs responsible for tuberculosis, bubonic plague, diphtheria, typhoid fever, pneumonia and the most dreaded of all - cholera.

Cholera Strikes Chicago

When Dr. Danforth arrived in Chicago in 1866, he found a city battling a cholera epidemic. The deadly scourge struck in the summer and fatalities increased steadily until October, when frightened citizens staged protest riots against the negligent economies of the city council.

Ironically, during the previous year, the city council had appointed the highly respected Dr. Nathan Smith Davis as chairman of a committee to investigate Chicago's sanitary conditions—overcrowded housing, inadequate sewers, and the dumping of garbage. City officials had attempted to implement the committee's recommendations, but the disease struck before they could take effect.

In 1867 a permanent seven-member Board of Health including three physicians was appointed by the mayor and judges of the Superior Court.[2] By the end of 1868, the new board had inaugurated inspection of slaughterhouses, the city's sewerage system had been greatly extended and 230,000 of Chicago's 241,000 inhabitants had been vaccinated against smallpox. In the following year milk inspection began, vaccination of all

---

[1] *Dr. Fenger helped reorganize the Passavant medical staff in 1885 and became medical staff president in 1895*

[2] *J. H. Rauch, Sanitary History of Chicago*

children was required and removal of epidemic patients to contagious disease hospitals was enforced.[1]

AND THEN CAME THE FIRE

"Soon after my appointment at St. Luke's in 1870," Dr. Danforth recalled in his memoirs, "I began to receive applications from Methodist friends, especially pastors of the city churches, for admission of charity cases to the small Episcopal hospital. As every staff member was permitted to admit charity patients, I soon found myself overburdened with requests, many of which I was obliged to refuse...My inability to help these sick poor awakened me keenly to the necessity of a Methodist hospital...

"Then, on October 8, 1871, came the Great Chicago Fire which destroyed a large portion of the city and left thousands homeless and destitute; hundreds sick, wounded, burned or prostrated by excitement and exposure...No one who followed the track of that fire all night, as I did, can ever forget those dreadful hours of devastation and horror.

"The pressure upon hospitals immediately became acute and intense. I was besieged with applications for admission to St. Luke's, not a fraction of which I could respond to. But we opened a temporary hospital in the lecture room and class rooms of the Centenary Church, and I spent most of my time for the following two or three weeks attending to the burned, the scalded, the wounded and sick people to whom we gave refuge. As soon as possible the authorities erected temporary barracks to which the homeless were transferred."

Other reports of the fire's aftermath painted an even darker picture than Dr. Danforth's portrayal. Six hospitals and medical schools were burned to the ground. They included Alexian Brothers, a hospital for men which traced its origin to the black plague of the 13th century; Chicago Hospital for Women and Children; Deaconess Hospital, later to become Passavant Memorial Hospital; Jewish Hospital, forerunner of Michael Reese; the clinical dispensary of Rush Medical College, and the Woman's Medical College. Among the few survivors were Cook County, St. Luke's and Mercy hospitals, and the Chicago Medical College.

[1]*Herman N. Bundesen, M.D., One Hundred Years of Public Health*

The Board of Health was credited with doing a herculean job of protecting the desolate citizenry. About 93,000 homeless people were crowded into the barracks which were inspected daily by sanitation officers. Physicians voluntarily staffed the temporary hospitals in churches and schoolhouses as well as the conveniently located dispensaries for ambulatory patients. Relief supplies were issued to the needy only on condition that they be vaccinated against smallpox. Yet despite the safeguards, more than 2,000 persons contracted smallpox in 1872. About a fourth of them died and the mortality among children was the highest ever recorded in Chicago.[1]

Although many Chicago physicians had lost all their worldly goods, they were seen rushing from shelter to shelter treating the sick. There were no lights, ditches were filled with debris, the water supply was polluted and sanitation entirely disrupted. A terrible filth and disorder prevailed.

When a semblance of order had been achieved, Dr. Danforth's efforts returned to his abiding interest. "By this time I was thoroughly aroused to the imperative and acute necessity for a Methodist hospital and I began to 'talk hospital' to Methodists whenever and wherever opportunity offered."

The doctor's persuasions were unproductive at that time, although a few spasmodic ripples of enthusiasm for a hospital surfaced now and then. Once the Chicago Methodist preachers even appointed a committee chaired by Robert M. Hatfield, D.D., father of Marcus P. Hatfield, M.D., to study the hospital question. However, the committee did not reply to Dr. Danforth's repeated inquiries or make its report known.

EASTERNERS SET SITES

Chicago had grown from a frontier town to a vigorous metropolis by 1881, just ten years after the fire. The Great Fire which leveled the city in 1871 halted only momentarily the city's phenomenal industrial and commercial expansion. The city's strategic location had attracted newcomers who added manpower and increased trade.

Adventurous and far-sighted men from the East had invested in the sparsely settled West and were ready to help develop the new area. One of these was William Deering, who came to Chicago in 1873 to engage in the

---

[1]*Herman N. Bundesen, M.D., One Hundred Years of Public Health*

manufacture of a harvester and automatic grain binder which would revolutionize agriculture throughout the world. William Deering was born in 1826 of a Puritan family in South Paris, Maine. He was educated in the Readfield Seminary in Maine and began the study of medicine under a Doctor Barrows of Fryeburg. His father, president of a woolen mill, needed William's assistance so the young man postponed his medical studies, presumably for a year. He remained in business and never resumed the study of medicine. However, the desire to be a physician influenced his philanthropies which were to dictate the destiny of Wesley Hospital.

In 1849 Deering was married to Abby Reed Barbour who died in 1856 leaving a son, Charles, who was graduated with distinction from the U.S. Naval Academy. William Deering later married Clara Cummings Hamilton and they had two children, a son, James, and daughter, Abby, who married Richard F. Howe. The Deering family moved to Evanston, Illinois, where James attended the Northwestern University preparatory school and later the Massachusetts Institute of Technology.

DEERING: FEEDING THE MULTITUDES

By 1879 William Deering had become the sole manufacturer of the Marsh harvester, a machine on which two men rode to cut and bind grain which previously had required six men following the reaper on foot. The new device was one of the first great steps in the evolution of mechanically harvested grain.

In 1901 Deering became ill and retired from active business leaving his two sons and son-in-law, who had become partners, in charge of the company. In the following year, the Deering Harvester Company merged with the International Harvester Company headed by Cyrus Hall McCormick. The Expanded International Harvester Company represented almost 85 percent of the world's farm machinery business.

William Deering's health was restored and he began to spend much of his time at his home in Coconut Grove, near Miami, Florida. He was a devout member of the Methodist Church and his support of its work covered the wide breadth of the church activities. Because of his profound interest in medicine he directed his attention to Northwestern University where his friend, Dr. Nathan Smith Davis, was bringing about reforms in medical education. How these interests came together to assure the growth of a Methodist hospital will unfold in later pages.

SWIFT: MEAT FOR THE WORLD

The meat packing industry also was pertinent to Chicago's growth and health in the 1870s. Although the established Western meat dealers, Nelson Morris and Philip D. Armour, took measures to abide by City Council health regulations, 72 other slaughterhouses and 281 rendering tanks had no apparatus to deter the fetid gases which generated from the stockyard. Infected meat was being sold for food and established safety measures were not being enforced.[1]

A solution was provided through the ingenuity of Gustavus Franklin Swift, another Easterner who came to Chicago. Swift introduced the refrigerator car, which insured Chicago's dominance in the meat packing industry. According to *The Yankee of the Yards*, G. F. Swift's biography by his son, Louis F. Swift, "The improvements in sanitation and the development of inspection methods constituted one of G. F. Swift's notable contributions to the preparation of meats for human consumption. His methods, worked out in the light of scientific discoveries, formed a basis for the inspection and control exercised by the Bureau of Animal Industry of the United States Government."

Gustavus Franklin Swift was born in Cape Cod Village, Maine, in 1839, and moved to Chicago in 1875. Already a successful meat wholesaler, he began slaughtering cattle in Chicago and sending edible parts east in refrigerated cars.

In 1880 Gustavus and his brother, Edwin C., became partners and the company was incorporated as Swift & Company with $300,000 capital stock. In less than three years, it increased to $3,000,000, then on and on to $25,000,000. Within 15 years Swift & Company had branches in every strategic city in the United States, with quantities of meat transported in refrigerated ships to outlets throughout Europe.

In 1861, Franklin Gustavus Swift had married Annie Maria Higgins who, with nine of their eleven children, survived him. He died at age 64 of an internal hemorrhage following an operation. Thrifty, industrious and

[1]*Lewis and Smith, The Tenements of Chicago, 1936*

rigidly honest, Swift had one other interest besides his family and business: his church. The Swifts were extremely active and benevolent in all interests of the Methodist Episcopal Church, especially those pertaining to the establishment and growth of a hospital in Chicago. This development was to become a noble family tradition which descendants[1] faithfully carried on.

PROBLEMS OF GROWTH

Chicago was proud of its increasing prominence in world trade, but the new metropolis was dangerously lacking in some areas. Thousands of immigrants had arrived to work in the stockyards and the factories, and to man the new agricultural machines. This large-scaled population influx produced dangerous overcrowding in slum areas. Small houses built for single families housed a family in each room.

Although attempts had been made to control the grosser sanitary abuses, the city's growth and the prevalence of epidemic disease were directly related. In 1894 the United States commissioner of labor reported that sanitary conditions were worse in Chicago than in New York, Philadelphia or Baltimore.

THE CHILDREN SUFFERED MOST

Children had the smallest chance for survival. By 1871, the mortality rate among Chicago children rose to 70.7 percent. They accounted for over half of all deaths in the city. Many were children of the foreign-born who lived in the undrained section of the city. The ignorance and illiteracy of their parents, unable to follow instructions of clinics and hospitals, made matters worse. Chicago did take steps to provide cleanliness, quarantine and pure water as advocated by its physicians. But public support, funds, manpower and knowledge could not nearly meet the need. However, during the period of Chicago's greatest growth, which occurred between 1855 and 1895, the mortality rate was actually reduced and no outbreak of cholera or typhoid took the toll of earlier years.

[1]*Edward F. Swift III, great grandson of G. F. Swift, was chairman of the Wesley Board of Trustees in 1972 when the Hospital merged with Passavant. He was elected the first chairman of the Board of Directors of the newly-formed Northwestern Memorial Hospital.*

HOPE LIES AHEAD

Chicago women still faced the grave danger of childbed fever prevalent the world over in the 19th century. The likelihood of puerperal contagion increased in the crowded city where births usually occurred in unclean tenement apartments.

The day was not far away, however, when physicians would insist upon fresh air and sunlight, good ventilation, adequate sewerage and aseptic obstetrical procedures as disease-preventing measures. That day would coincide with the founding of Wesley Hospital in 1888.

How Wesley Began   Chapter 2

D r. Danforth's unrelenting efforts to establish a Methodist hospital were to meet success through an unexpected source. On October 20, 1885, under the aegis of the Methodist Church, the Chicago Training School for City, Home and Foreign Missions opened its doors on the city's near north side. "The founders of this institution, beyond all question," Dr. Danforth wrote, "were Josiah Shelley Meyer and his paragon of a wife, Lucy Rider Meyer. They worked unceasingly and unfalteringly, and after many discouragements, success crowned their efforts."

Lucy Jane Rider, a graduate of Oberlin College in Ohio, had taken medical courses at Philadelphia and had received an honorary doctorate in medicine from the Women's Medical College of Chicago. She was a Methodist field worker and became concerned that no school in the United States offered training to women for missionary work. She convinced such prominent Methodists as Dr. Danforth, William Deering, Norman Wait Harris and the Reverend Matthew M. Parkhurst, of this need.

Miss Rider was field secretary of the Illinois State Sunday School Association when she met Josiah Shelley Meyer, administrative assistant of the Chicago Young Men's Christian Association. They were married May 21, 1885. He had trained at Northwestern (now McCormick) Theological Seminary, as well as at a commercial school and had worked in a newspaper office. It is said that the talents of each of these two leaders so supplemented those of the other that it would have been impossible for so preeminent a success to have been achieved without the work of either one.

Mrs. Meyer addressed a Chicago Methodist Preachers' meeting June 15, 1885, demonstrating to the assembly that a training school for missionaries was essential, and she induced the ministers to adopt at once "measures to establish such an institution." Her impassioned speech gained full support of the clergy and it began the life work of the Meyers. Through the Chicago Training School for City, Home and Foreign Missions and through its students, forty institutions - for orphans, the elderly, the homeless, sick and injured - were founded during the lifetimes of Lucy Rider and Josiah Shelley Meyer.

The school opened October 20, 1885, in an "old-fashioned house at 19 Park Street with two stories and a basement swell front," and was soon overflowing with students. The charter obtained from the State of Illinois June 24, 1886, named the following Trustees: William E. Blackstone, Dr. Isaac N. Danforth, William Deering, George D. Elderkin, James B. Hobbs, the Reverend Matthew M. Parkhurst, Charles E. Simmons, Hiram J. Thompson and Joseph L. Whitlock. Bylaws were adopted June 29, 1886, and the following were elected officers: The Reverend Parkhurst, president; Mr. Whitlock, vice president; Mrs. Meyer, secretary, and the Reverend Meyer, business secretary. In addition to the trustees and officers, the executive committee included Mrs. Danforth, Mrs. Robert D. Fowler, Mrs. Hobbs, and Mrs. E. E. Marcy.

The house on Park Street soon proved to be wholly inadequate so the trustees purchased a desirable lot at the northwest corner of Dearborn Avenue and Ohio Street. The school took possession of its own building at 114 Dearborn Avenue December 8, 1886. Mrs. Meyer wrote in her book, *Deaconesses*, published in 1889, "There was not a knob on a door nor a particle of paint on any portion . . . The odor of paint gave flavor to our classroom exercises for many a week." As Mrs. Meyer worked with the students, she found they often were called upon to tend the sick, desperately needing help in their homes. It was obvious that studies in nursing should be added to the curriculum.

Now Then, Do It

Mrs. Meyer's enterprises were generally considered "prophetic" because of their immediate success and rapid growth. In 1887 she initiated another project, a Home for Deaconesses. The idea had developed in the training school's religious class where much had been said of Phoebe, Paul's "helper of many," and the deaconesses of the early church (see Prologue, footnote[1], page xiv). In the June 1887 issue of *Message*, a Methodist monthly publication, Mrs. Meyer announced the opening of a deaconess home within the training school during the summer months. "In this home we propose to receive such ladies as shall be approved, who wish to devote themselves to city missionary work," she explained. "We believe that a headquarters for missionaries may be a seed with a life-germ in it. It may be small, but so was the mustard seed."

A progress report in the October *Message* by Mrs. Meyer disclosed, "The favorite motto of the training school has been the words of Abner to the Elders of Israel: 'Now then, do it.'[1] And we have done it!" The work of the deaconesses became a recognized part of the church program.

The first Methodist deaconesses in America were Isabelle Reeves, Fannie Canfield and Evelyn Keeler who were licensed and consecrated in June, 1889, at Centenary Church in Chicago. Mrs. Meyer, whose services to the training school were on a volunteer basis (as were those of her husband), became the first woman to wear the simple black uniform of the American Methodist deaconess.

DEACONESS NURSES REINFORCE DANFORTH EFFORTS

Dr. Danforth recalled in his memoirs "Both my wife and myself were greatly interested in the work of the deaconesses," adding "although I am perfectly safe in saying that her judgment and counsel were regarded as far more valuable than mine, an opinion with which I joyfully concur.

"But during all this time, my dreams of a Methodist hospital haunted me with increasing fervor...From the very beginning of the training school movement, the Meyers, husband and wife, and myself had conferences on the hospital question...In the summer of 1888 the plan of having a class of 'Nurse Deaconesses' was adopted. It seemed to clarify the atmosphere and provide for the important matter of supplying nurses for

[1]*Samuel 3:18 The motto later became a motivating force for action by members of the Wesley Ladies Aid Association*

the hospital on the one hand; on the other hand of providing training and experience which the nurse deaconesses must have."

A three-story building next to the training school was given by Mrs. A. M. Smith of Oak Park, Illinois, to provide improved living quarters for twelve deaconesses eager to become nurses. Dr. Danforth appraised the situation and decided that three or four of the rooms in the Smith annex could be used for clinical work. So, with rooms for patients, deaconesses for nurses, and Dr. Danforth and colleagues for physicians, the time had come to start a hospital. "All we needed was financial and moral support," Dr. Danforth asserted, " and that came about quite providentially."

The Firmament Showeth His Handiwork

"It is not stretching the truth," Dr. Danforth relates in his memoirs, "to say that Wesley Hospital was heralded by the flash of lightning and the roar of heaven's artillery."

The Danforth family was staying at its summer cottage at Lake Bluff in August, 1888, when their neighbors, Mr. and Mrs. Robert D. Fowler, came to call on Sunday afternoon. As they prepared to leave, torrents of rain fell, lightning flashed and thunder roared like firearms exploding. The Fowlers remained at the Danforths until the terrible thunderstorm abated.

"I knew Mr. Fowler well," Dr. Danforth confided. "He was one of the noblest men in Chicago Methodism. He was liberal in all things; gave freely of his wealth for all good purposes; was ever ready with his counsel in furthering works of charity, and he was never happier than when engaged in some work for the relief of the sick and suffering.

"I thought about the hospital enterprise and wondered whether I could engage the interest of this splendid Englishman in it. I knew he was constantly besieged by charitable solicitations but the falling rain, streaks of lightning and thunderbolts seeemed to unite in urging me to use the opportunity that might not be offered again.

"And so, much in doubt, I broached the subject to Mr. Fowler. I was greatly gratified at his response. It was decided that afternoon to begin immediately employing the services and facilities of the Training School for City, Home and Foreign Missions; and the affiliated Deaconess Home, permitting students of the latter to gain the practical training to fit them for their chosen work as nurses."

In less than a week a small group including, in addition to Dr. Danforth and Mr. Fowler, Harlow N. Higinbotham, partner of Marshall Field; the Reverend Luke Hitchcock and the Reverend C. G. Trusdell, presiding elder of the Chicago Methodist district, met to arrange an organizational meeting. Their signatures appeared on the following letter sent to civic and business leaders, clergymen and others who might be interested in founding a Methodist hospital.

Dear Sir:

For some years past the necessity for a Methodist Hospital in Chicago has been recognized by those most concerned with the needs of the sick poor. It seems to the undersigned that the time for action has come. We therefore earnestly invite you to attend a meeting of the friends of the movement at the Sherman House club rooms on Saturday evening, September 8 at 8 o'clock. The chief arguments in favor of the immediate action follow:

First, the hospital is a necessity; the honor of our denomination and the equities of the case demand it. Our sick poor are cared for by the hospitals operated and supported by other denominations and we have already incurred obligations that should not be increased.

Second, the pupils in our Training School for City, Home and Foreign Missions, and in our Deaconesses Home, all require observation and experience to fit them for their particular work. Nothing else can supply this want. Both missionaries and deaconesses will be thrown much among the sick; in fact, the work of the latter will be primarily the care of the sick and helpless. A hospital should be organized in connection with the Training School and Deaconesses Home. We do not favor a large or costly building, but we do recommend the immediate organization of a small hospital in a portion of the training school buildings which, we are informed, can be obtained for this purpose. The advantages of this plan are obvious. It furnishes a refuge for the sick poor, it offers clinical facilities to our students and they in turn will take entire charge of the nursing service.

Believing that you will recognize the necessity for this movement and will give it your personal and financial support, we urge you to attend the conference at the time and place above indicated.

Very truly yours,

Fourteen persons answered the call and met at the Sherman House on the evening of September 8. The original five were augmented by the Reverend Josiah Shelley Meyer, Dr. Marcus P. Hatfield, Judge Edmund W. Burke, Charles Busby, Mr. and Mrs. James B. Hobbs, Dr. B. W. Griffin, James

Harvey and George D. Elderkin. It was decided that a hospital be established following the plan advocated by Dr. Danforth, namely: in a small way in temporary quarters provided by the training school and deaconess home.

What's in a Name?

The high hopes of the founders of the infant institution were reflected in the lengthy discussion concerning its name. This was first on the agenda at the second meeting on September 26, 1888. "Methodist Episcopal Hospital" and other polysyllable names were objectionable to Mr. Higinbotham because long and compound names were likely to lead to litigation over legacies. A slight error in writing the name could furnish an opportunity for displeased heirs-at-law to attempt to break wills in which the hospital would be a legatee. To prevent such problems, James Hart Manny, inventor associated with Cyrus H. McCormick and later William Deering, proposed "Wesley Hospital." The simple name in honor of John Wesley, the enlightened religious leader and physician who had started free dispensaries in 18th century England, was adopted by the group.

The Board of Trustees and the Charter

The group attending the second meeting also elected thirty members of the Board of Trustees and drew up the petition for a charter.

The petition was signed by the entire Board of Trustees: Abraham H. Benson; Lester L. Bond, lawyer and two-term member of the Illinois State Legislature; William E. Blackstone; Frank M. Bristol, D.D., Bishop of the Methodist Church, 1908-1924; Edmund W. Burke, lawyer, judge of the Cook County Circuit Court for nine years; Charles Busby; Isaac N. Danforth, M.D., nationally known physician; William Deering, president of Deering Harvester Company until it merged with International Harvester; David R. Dyche, M.D., founder of the Illinois College of Pharmacy, president of Citizen's League of Evanston which enforced a prohibitory liquor law; Charles B. Eggleston, president of Flour Grain and Provision Company, director of the Chicago Stock Exchange; George E. Elderkin; Josiah M. Fleming; Horace A. Goodrich, real estate executive; Robert D. Fowler, retired capitalist; Norman W. Harris, president of the Harris Trust and Savings Bank of Chicago; James S. Harvey; Marcus P. Hatfield, pediatrician and author of books on children's diseases; Luke Hitchcock,

D.D.; Matson Hill; James B. Hobbs, retired merchant; Emanuel Honsinger, D.D.S.; Oliver W. Horton, lawyer, Circuit Court judge, 1887-1903; Henry G. Jackson, D.D., pastor of the Centenary Church in Chicago; Charles E. Manderville, D.D.; William H. Rand, president of Rand, McNally & Company; Robert D. Sheppard, D.D., professor of history and political economy at Northwestern University; Hiram J. Thompson; Charles G. Trusdell, D.D., superintendent of the Chicago Relief and Aid Society, presiding elder of the Chicago district, Methodist Episcopal Church; James L. Whitlock; and Milton H. Wilson, board chairman, wholesale men's furnishings.

Wesley Hospital began existence as a legal entity upon receipt of the Charter:

State of Illinois
Department of State
Henry D. Dement, Secretary of State
To all to whom these presents shall come, Greeting

Whereas, a Certificate, duly signed and acknowledged, having been filed in the Office of the Secretary of State on the 26th day of October, A.D. 1888, for the organization of Wesley Hospital, under and in accordance with the provisions of "An Act Concerning Corporations," approved April 18th, 1872, and in force July 1st, 1872, and all acts amendatory thereof, a copy of which Certificate is hereto attached:

Now Therefore, I, Henry D. Dement, Secretary of State of the State of Illinois, by virtue of the powers and duties vested in me by law, do hereby certify that the said Wesley Hospital is a legally organized corporation under the laws of this State.

In Testimony whereof, I hereto set my hand, and cause to be affixed the great Seal of the State. Done at the City of Springfield this twenty-sixth day of October, in the year of our Lord one thousand eight hundred and eighty-eight, and of the independence of the United States the one hundred and thirteenth.

(Seal)

Henry D. Dement
Secretary of State.

Dr. Danforth reported that the charter was filed for the records on October 27, 1888, and that Harlow N. Higinbotham defrayed the costs.

OFFICERS AND EXECUTIVE COMMITTEE

Organization of the board was continued at a meeting November 10 when Luke Hitchcock, D.D. was elected president, and Marcus P. Hatfield, M.D., secretary. Executive Committee members appointed were Isaac N. Danforth, M.D., David R. Dyche, M.D., Charles G. Trusdell, D.D., Hiram J. Thompson, James L. Whitlock, and George D. Elderkin, chairman.

The executive committee met for the first time in the parlors of the Grand Pacific Hotel on Tuesday, November 13 when a committee to draft a constitution and bylaws was appointed. Dr. Danforth called attention to the records of this meeting "chiefly because they show the infinitesimal beginnings of an enterprise which has now (1909) grown to such stalwart proportions."

NURSES AND ROOMS AVAILABLE

During a Ways and Means discussion, it was stated that five or six beds for patients were available at the training school until May 1, 1889. The school specified that suitable accommodations be provided deaconess nurses who would be dispossessed by the patients admitted. After May 1 twelve rooms could be obtained at the same location at a cost of $600 and the lodging of nurses employed.

Attached to the minutes was a document in the handwriting of Lucy Rider Meyer, principal of the Training School for Home and Foreign Missions, 114-122 Dearborn Avenue, on the school's letterhead which listed, in addition to Mrs. Meyer, James B. Hobbs, president; Mrs. Isaac N. Danforth, vice president; William E. Blackstone, secretary; George D. Elderkin, treasurer, and J. Shelley Meyer, business superintendent. The overlapping of the boards of the school and Wesley Hospital assured a close relationship. The document outlined the responsibilities of the training school in providing deaconess nurses for the hospital and the responsibility of the hospital in training the nurses and subsidizing their expenses.

OTHER OFFERS

At the next meeting, November 27, 1888, the executive committee met with three physicians representing the faculty of the Women's Medical College of Chicago. They offered a medical board to provide all the medical and surgical service of the hospital and to give the medical teaching necessary to train nurses. They also offered the ground and buildings then used for college purposes. The matter was held in abeyance several months, then dropped by both parties.

Another cooperative proposition was offered December 7 by Dr. J. R. Kewley of the Lakeside Sanitarium of Chicago where sick babies were given care during the summer months. Dr. Kewley offered property on the Lincoln Park lake shore free, on condition that its work be continued. This too was discussed and rejected. In the comments that followed the two affiliation proposals, it developed that Northwestern University also had an eye on Wesley Hospital.

The constitution and bylaws were drafted by L. L. Bond, O. H. Horton and Edmund W. Burke and were adopted by the Board of Trustees on January 5, 1889.

THE BIRTH OF WESLEY HOSPITAL

On the premise that a hospital exists only when it begins to admit patients, Wesley Hospital was born December 25, 1888. "On that eventful day while the Christmas bells were ringing," Dr. Danforth recalled in his writings, "Mrs. Hattie Dewar was driven in a cab to the Training School for City, Home and Foreign Missions at Dearborn and Ohio where we had arranged to receive a few patients temporarily. We find on the hospital record: *"Name*—Mrs. Hattie Dewar/*Physician*—Dr. I. N. Danforth/*Disease* —Inflammatory Rheumatism/*Discharged*—Cured February 7, 1889."[1]

Mrs. Meyer recalled in her book, *Deaconesses,* that "they were just finishing Christmas dinner when the doorbell rang. The patient was in such pain that she could not walk and Mr. Meyer helped carry her in."

Two other patients were admitted in early January and the constant care caused interruption of class schedules and other inconveniences to the training school. It was imperative that the patients be moved to appropriate quarters.

---

[1] *A letter from J. Shelley Meyer dated April 8, 1909 to Dr. Danforth states that the first patient was received on Thanksgiving, 1889. Dr. Danforth refuted the statement indicating that Meyer's memory had erred. The hospital records verify December 25, 1888 as the date on which Wesley's first patient was admitted.*

A house "suitable for hospital purposes at 355 East Ohio Street near Pine Avenue (now Michigan Avenue)" was reported available at a joint meeting of the executive committee and Board of Trustees January 19, 1889. A sum of $2,000 was pledged to pay the monthly rent of $65. Mr. Elderkin, Dr. Dyche and Dr. Danforth were appointed as a special committee authorized to "hire a building and begin hospital work as soon as possible."

A Modest Start
Chapter 3

Wesley Hospital's first home, an unpretentious three-story and basement annex structure, had only one qualification for admitting patients: its proximity to the deaconess nurse training school at 114 Dearborn Avenue. According to Dr. Danforth, the house was "thoroughly out of repair and sadly in need of a scrubber and decorator."

On February 1, 1889, Mrs. Dewar and the other patients were moved from the deaconess home to Wesley Hospital at 355 East Ohio Street. The building contained 12 rooms with 14 patient beds, nurses' quarters and utility facilities. Although the patient capacity was increased, there still was no provision for male patients.

Miss E. J. McBurnie, a deaconess nurse, was appointed superintendent of nurses; Miss A. E. Cox, matron and housekeeper; and Josiah Shelley Meyer became warden and chaplain. These appointments complied with a contract between the Chicago Deaconess Home and Wesley Hospital accepted February 27, 1889, stipulating that:

(1) the home provide all nursing and housekeeping personnel required and that the service follow the rules and regulations of both the Home and the Hospital.

(2) the personnel receive only the support given other members of the Deaconess Home. In each case, persons provided by the Home must first be accepted by the Hospital Executive Committee and the Medical Staff before entering service.

(3) the agreement may be revoked at any time by either party after 90 days notice.

Item 2 referred to regulations for members of the Deaconess Home which stated "they will receive no salary, but we promise them a home and board as the Lord may provide, and the payment of necessary carfare." Under this arrangement, neither the superintendent of nurses, the matron nor student nurses were to receive pay for their services. "However beautiful in theory," Dr. Danforth commented later, "the plan proved to be infeasible in practice and it was the beginning of a great deal of trouble, misunderstanding and friction in the following ten years.

WESLEY'S FIRST BABY

The first baby to be born in Wesley Hospital was due to arrive in mid March, 1889. The expectant parents, Mr. and Mrs. Lentz; the nurses, in fact, the entire hospital population, had unanimously agreed that the child should be named John Wesley Lentz. But when the infant was delivered on March 18, nature had decreed (according to a deaconess' decorous note) that "John" was inappropriate. There was a hasty switch and the baby girl was named Susanna Wesley Lentz honoring the mother of the famous churchman for whom the Hospital was named.

MEDICAL STAFF APPOINTED

The appointment of the Medical Staff was the major item on the agenda for the meeting of the Board of Trustees at the Sherman House on March 20. The first Medical Staff of Wesley Hospital consisted of:

Consulting Staff - Nathan S. Davis, M.D., L.L.D., internist; William H. Byford, M.D., internist; E. O. F. Roler, M.D., obstetrician; S. C. Blake, M.D., neurologist; and Reuben Ludlam, A.M., M.D., homeopathic physician.

Attending Staff - Isaac N. Danforth, A.M., M.D., pathologist and internist; Marcus P. Hatfield, M.D., pediatrician; Charles W. Earle, M.D., obstetrician; and F. C. Schaefer, M.D., surgeon.

Interns - Ross Engleman, M.D. and Flora Lorman, M.D.

At a later meeting, Marie Mergler, M.D. was appointed gynecologist. Dr. Danforth was elected staff president and Dr. Hatfield, secretary. All appointees accepted their positions promptly except Dr. Davis whose characteristic reply was read by Dr. Hatfield at the April meeting of the Board of Trustees.

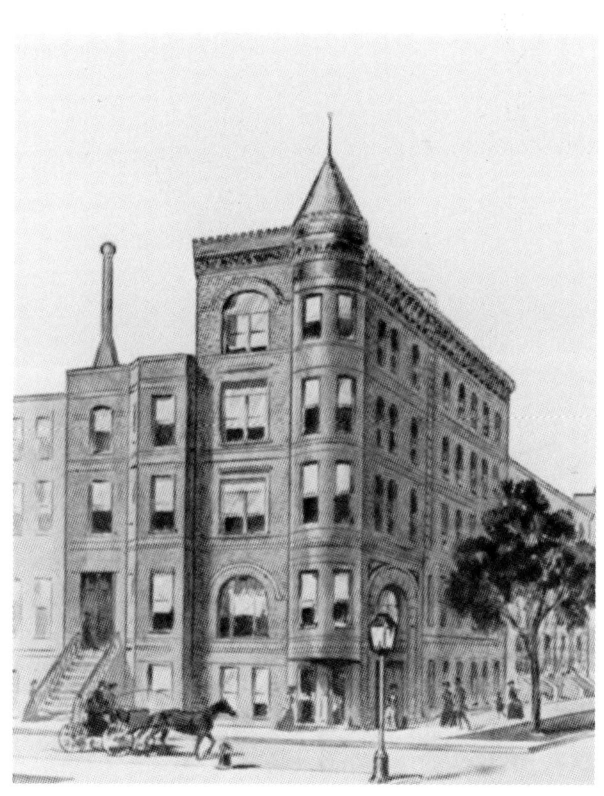

Wesley Hospital began on Christmas Day, 1888, in the Chicago Training School for City Home and Foreign Missions at the corner of Dearborn and Ohio streets.

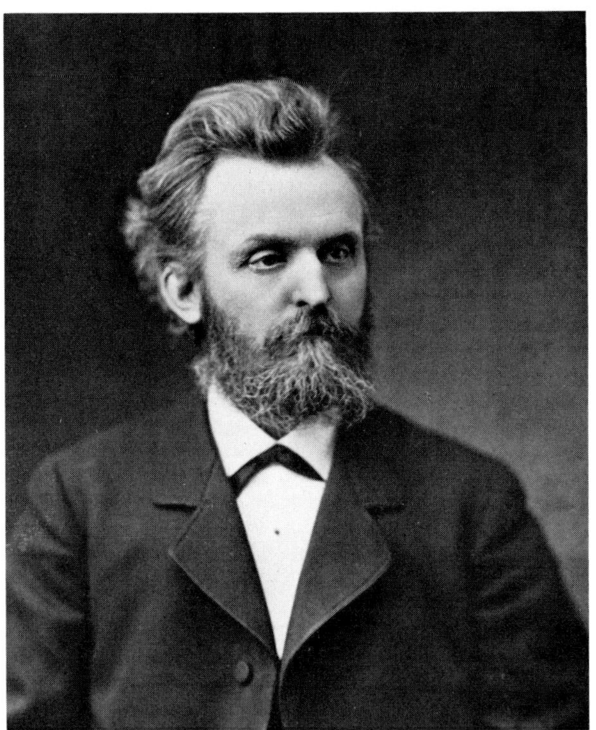

Courtesy of Chicago Historical Society

Issac Newton Danforth, M.D.,
1835-1911, was the founder of Wesley
Hospital and organizer of its medical staff.

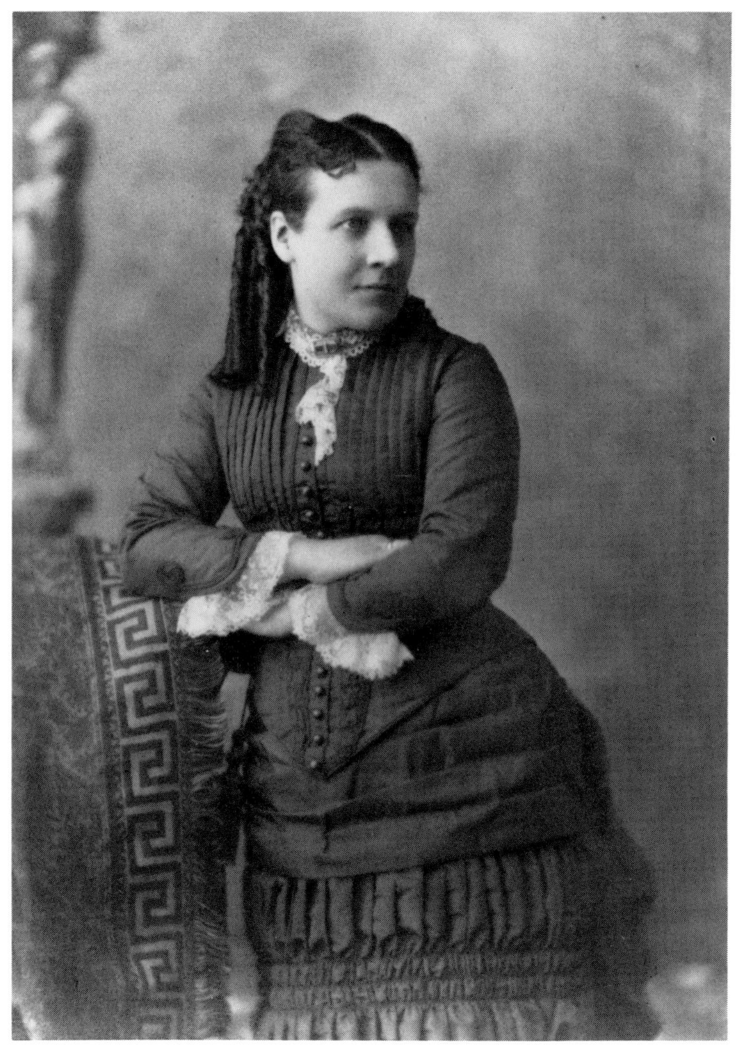

*Elizabeth Skelton Danforth established the
Wesley Ladies Aid Association in 1889 and
served as its first president.*

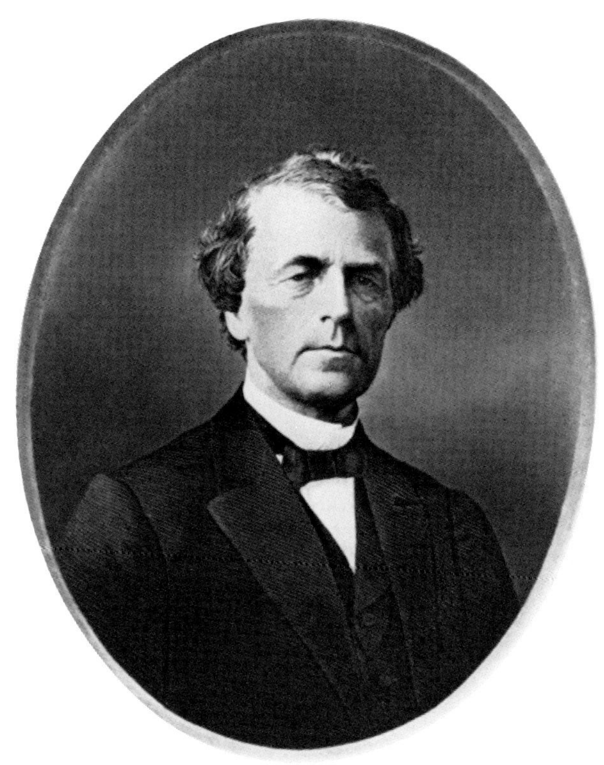

*Luke Hitchcock, D.D., born in Lebanon,
N.Y., in 1813, was elected first president of
the Wesley Board of Trustees in November, 1889.*

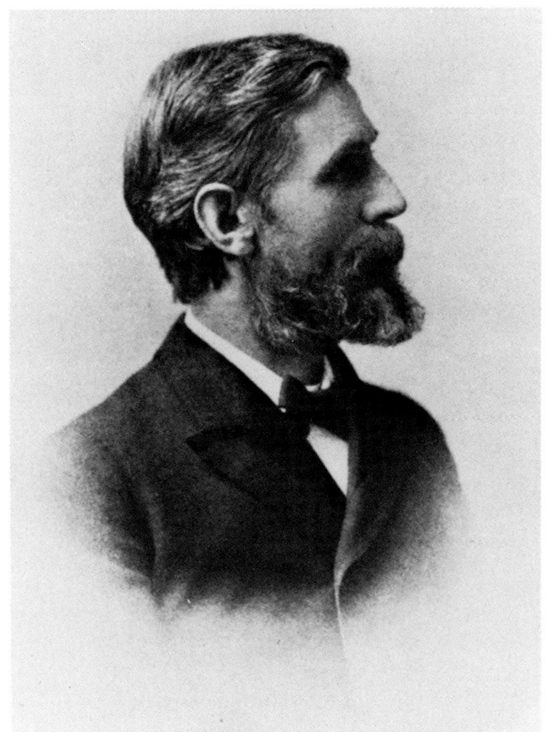

Courtesy of Field Museum

*Harlow N. Higinbotham, partner of Marshall
Field, arranged the hospital organizational
meeting held September 8, 1888.*

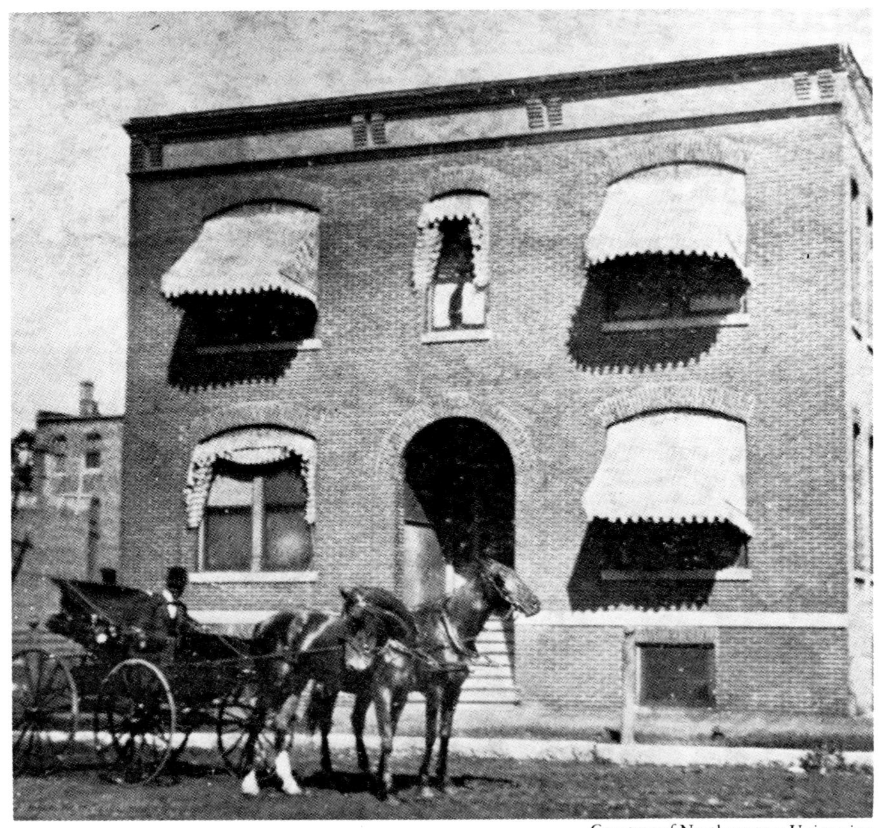

*Wesley's 35-bed building opened in 1891.
Next door, in 1893, Davis Hall arose with
amphitheater where surgical patients were
transported by stretcher for ten years.*

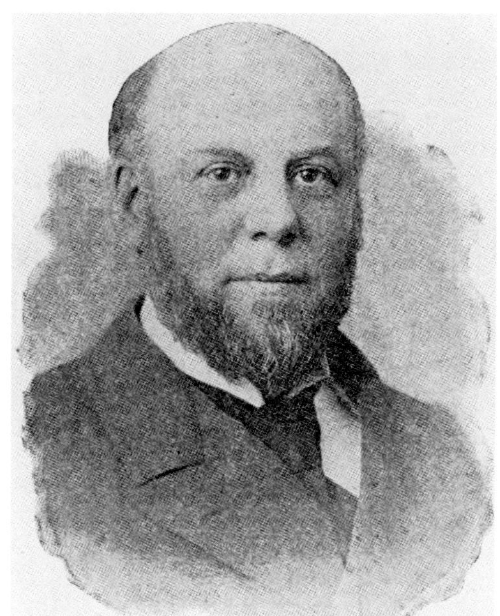

Courtesy of Harris Trust and Savings Bank

Norman Wait Harris, 1846-1916, charter board member, gave the residence for 80 nurses in 1906 and started the Deaconess Pension Fund with a liberal donation.

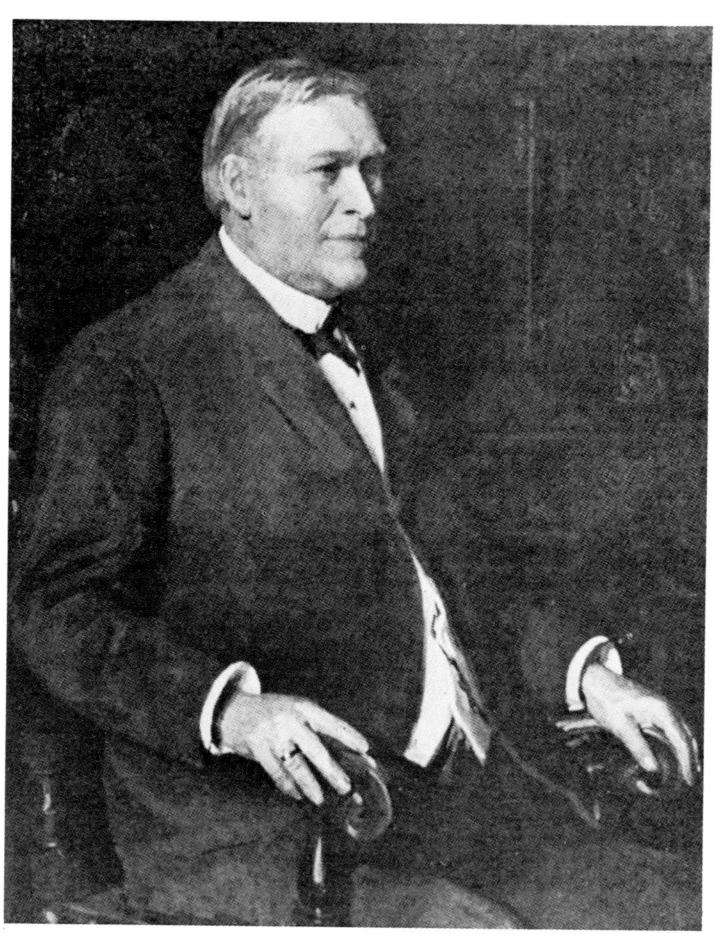

*Arthur Dixon, 1837-1917, came to
Chicago from Ireland in 1861. He joined
the Wesley board in 1899, first of an
unbroken line of Wesley trustees.*

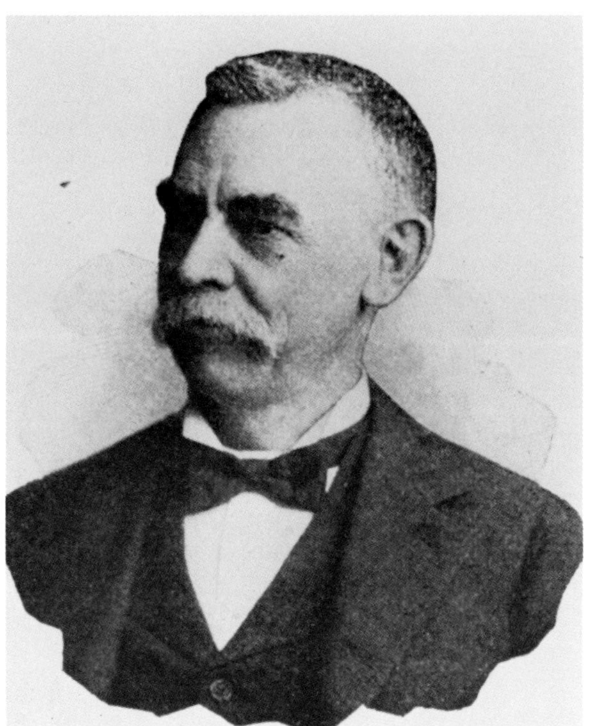

Courtesy of Iowa State Historical Society

*James S. Harvey, Jr., charter board
member, donated his services as
superintendent and treasurer, 1895-1901,
and cleared Wesley of its debt.*

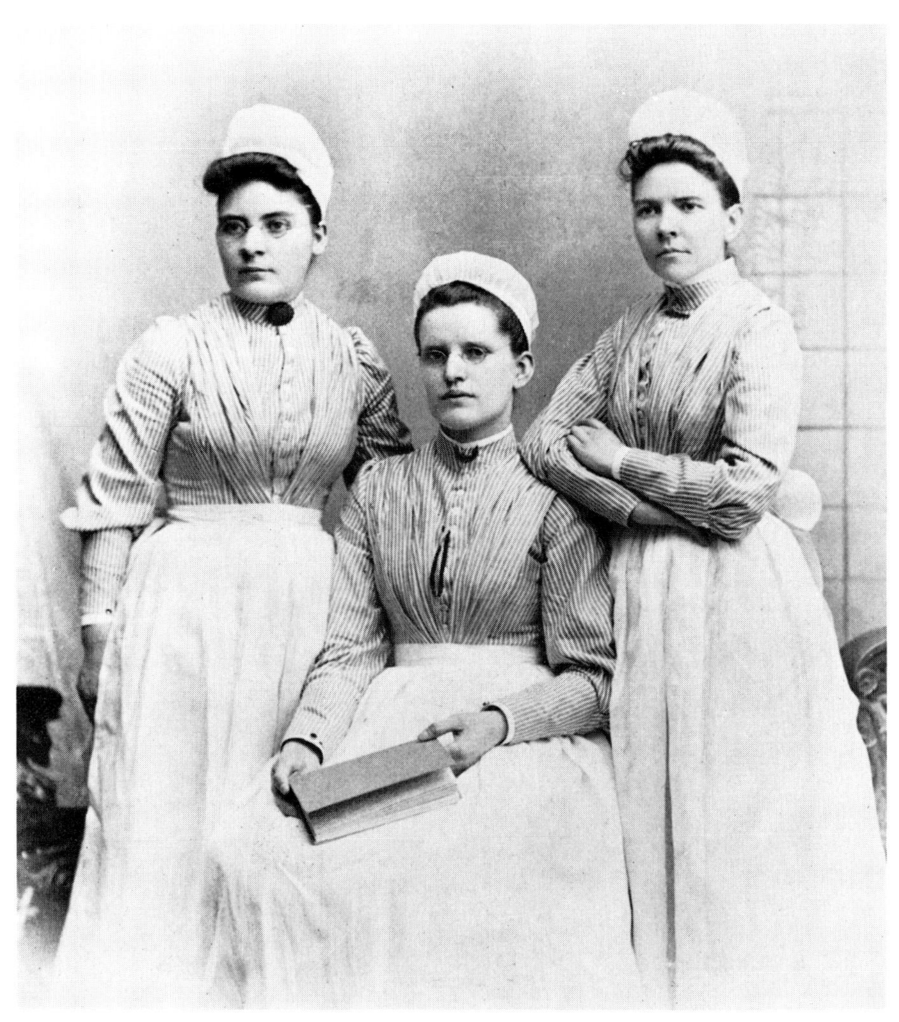

Wesley's first class of student nurses was graduated in 1890. From left: Margaret A. Cox, Elizabeth Calbeck and Emma A. Davis.

Dear Doctor:

Your kind note informing me that the Executive Committee of Wesley Hospital had elected me a member of the Consulting Staff of said hospital is received. If it is expected that members of the Consulting Staff shall be actually consulted in all matters relating to the medical and surgical management of the hospital, and in the treatment of such cases as may desire such counsel, I will accept the appointment, and will endeavor to discharge the appropriate duties of the position. But I am entirely unwilling to accept the position merely for the purpose of having my name go before the public as a member of the staff without any duties to perform.
With much respect.

Yours truly,
(signed)
N. S. Davis

Doctor Davis was assured that his appointment would be an active one as it proved to be a short time later. Drs. Danforth and Schaefer had agreed that an operation was necessary in the case of Bishop S. M. Merrill who was in Wesley with acute appendicitis. Dr. Davis was called in and he advised the attending physicians to wait a little and use "old-fashioned poulticing." They did; the inflammation subsided and did not return. The Bishop escaped an operation, lived a long life and carried his appendix to his grave.

Shortly after the incident, the sister of the Bishop's wife had an attack of acute appendicitis while visiting the Merrills. The Bishop, remembering his experience and the wisdom of Dr. Davis, tried "old-fashioned poulticing" on his sister-in-law. The consequence was a ruptured appendix with blood poisoning, peritonitis, a delayed operation and death. Dr. Davis pointed out that, in this case, "old-fashioned poulticing" cost a life which prompt surgery would have saved. Diagnosis and treatment were better left to physicians then, as now.

First Annual Report

When George D. Elderkin, chairman of the executive committee, presented his first annual report November 2, 1889, he stressed the crowded conditions and the need for more beds. During the year 90 patients had occupied the Hospital's 14 beds. Thirty patients paid from $3 to $10 per week; the remaining 60 were charity patients. The primitive working conditions were described: "The doctors performed operations in the wards permeated by the smell of scorched flannel. This was caused by nurses who sterilized water on the kitchen stove and carried it to the bedside in open pitchers. Bricks heated in the oven and wrapped in flannel kept the water hot during the surgical procedure."

The superintendent of nurses, Miss McBurnie, went to China for missionary work and was succeeded by Miss Mary E. Simonds under whom the first and second classes of nurses were graduated. The first one, the Class of 1890, was composed of Margaret A. Cox, Elizabeth Calbeck and Emma A. Davis, forerunners of more than a thousand Wesley graduates before the school was temporarily closed in 1935.

THE LADIES AID FORMED

Even before Wesley Hospital had received its charter, women were meeting in their churches planning ways to assist. The Ladies Aid Association of Wesley Hospital was organized on March 20, 1889, with Mrs. Isaac N. Danforth as president. Its constitution stated the purpose "to aid the Board of Trustees of Wesley Hospital and to secure the help of Methodism in the work of the Hospital."

Although minutes were not kept until October 9, 1900, Mrs. Henry G. Jackson, a charter member, described the first few months: "With almost no conveniences at hand, we women rallied to the call and soon had a society in good working order. Though not many were able to attend the regular monthly meetings, women from all the Methodist churches were quick to respond with contributions of money and necessary items such as bandages, bed linen, towels and infants' layettes."

At the end of its first year, the Ladies Aid Association had 147 members from 35 churches in the Rock River Conference.[1] The Sunday following June 17, the birthday anniversary of John Wesley, was proclaimed "Hospital Sunday" and all 371 churches in the Rock River Conference were asked to solicit donations for the struggling Wesley Hospital. Hospital Sunday became an annual event which fostered good will and obtained needed funds.

[1]*The term, Rock River Conference, refers to the organization of 371 Methodist churches in the northern section of Illinois including Chicago, its outlying areas, and smaller cities such as Joliet, Aurora, Dixon, Rockford and Waukegan.*

Wesley's Dilemma — Chapter 4

There were sharp differences of opinion in 1890 concerning the permanent location of Wesley Hospital. Friends of the Training School for Home and Foreign Missions, which provided nursing service and administration, favored property available on Ohio Street near the school and its deaconess home. Those who were more closely associated with Northwestern University were partial to property at the corner of 25th and Dearborn streets where the university planned to locate its professional schools.

A review of the development of the Chicago Medical College, Medical Department of Northwestern University, during the second half of the 19th century, will help explain Wesley's indecision in 1890. The impact of the medical college and its instigator, Dr. Nathan Smith Davis, had a definite bearing on the outcome.

In 1849, at the age of 32, Dr. Davis had moved from New York City, where he practiced and taught at the College of Physicians and Surgeons, to Chicago to be chairman of physiology and pathology at Rush Medical College. Believing that hospital experience is an intrinsic part of medical education, Dr. Davis established Mercy Hospital, chartered in 1852, where Rush students could gain clinical knowledge.

RETROGRESSION IN EDUCATION

A number of Rush faculty members, led by Dr. Davis, had become overtly dissatisfied with the failure of the president and trustees to improve the school by raising requirements for the degree of Doctor of Medicine. A relaxed pattern was prevalent at medical schools throughout the country. No stipulations concerning previous formal education were prescribed, the annual term was only 16 weeks, all subjects were taught simultaneously to first and second year students, and experience in dissecting was optional. It was said that medical education in 1855 was inferior to that of the earliest colonial medical schools.

In 1857, Dr. Davis, who had championed medical education improvement in New York and Chicago for 15 years, and Dr. William H. Byford, chairman of obstetrics at Rush and advocate of reforms, proposed a new curriculum at an informal meeting of the Rush faculty which would correct the inadequacies. However, the trustees, who feared that new policies might adversely affect enrollment, refused to adopt any change from the established curriculum.

ANOTHER PROPOSAL

During the discord of 1857, a charter was granted to another school, Lind University, named for Sylvester Lind, a benefactor who was in the lumber business. Located in Lake Forest and later named Lake Forest University, it began as a preparatory school with plans to become a college of liberal arts, then to acquire professional departments. This plan would have a significant influence on Northwestern University and ultimately on Wesley Hospital.

Dissident doctors at Rush agreed on the need for a medical school with sound educational principles better adapted to scientific and medical knowledge available at the time. Such principles did not exist in any medical school in mid 19th century America. The doctors knew that reform was not possible at Rush, so they agreed to talk with the executive committee of the new Lind University. The progressive views of Drs. Davis and Byford were shared by Drs. Edmund Andrews, Hosmer A. Johnson, Ralph N. Isham and David Rutter, all of whom participated in the preparatory negotiations. Lind University accepted the proposal which would revolutionize medical education.

After consideration the agreement was accepted and signed, establishing the Medical Department of Lind University. On March 24, the following officers were elected: Hosmer A. Johnson, M.D., president; Ralph N. Isham, M.D., recording secretary; William H. Byford, M.D., corresponding secretary; and Edmund Andrews, M.D., treasurer. Commenting on this period in his history of Northwestern University Medical School, Dr. Leslie B. Arey noted: "It is interesting and probably significant, that the ages of the active founders of this new enterprise ranged from 24 (Isham) to 42 (Davis); Dr. Rutter, often designated in historical reference as aged or well advanced in years, had just turned 58!"

Eleven professorships, about twice the number in other medical schools, were established. The professorial chairs and the faculty members who occupied them were: Descriptive Anatomy, Dr. Titus DeVille; Demonstrative Anatomy, Dr. Horace Wardner; Physiology and Histology, Dr. John H. Hollister; Surgical Anatomy and Operative Surgery, Dr. Ralph N. Isham; Principles and Practice of Surgery, Dr. Edmund Andrews; Principles and Practice of Medicine, Dr. Nathan S. Davis; Materia Medica and Therapeutics, Dr. Hosmer A. Johnson; Organic Chemistry and Toxicology, Dr. Frederick Mahla; General Pathology and Public Hygiene, Dr. M. K. Taylor; Medical Jurisprudence, Dr. Henry G. Spafford; Midwifery and Diseases of Women and Children, Dr. William H. Byford, and Dr. David Rutter, Emeritus Professor of Midwifery.

THE REFORMATION OF MEDICAL EDUCATION

Classes of the Medical Department of Lind University began October 9, 1859. The school opened on two floors of the five-story brick building on the northwest corner of Market (now Wacker) and Randolph streets in what was known as the Lind Block. Mercy Hospital, located on Wabash Avenue with 60 beds, provided clinical experience. This institution had transferred use of its facilities to the new school when its founder, Dr. Davis, resigned from Rush Medical College.

The efforts of the innovators were recognized in both the professional and lay press who apparently realized that a new era in medical education had begun. The student body increased steadily from 33 in 1859 to 81 in 1862. But the events in which the nation was embroiled were to involve the fledgling school.

The effects of the Civil War had destroyed the fortune of Sylvester Lind, who by 1863 was unable to fulfill his pledges to the Lind University. The medical faculty had no alternative but to accept the situation and seek new quarters. The members themselves authorized the purchase of a building at State Street near 22nd Street (now Cermak Road). They pledged to donate their lecture fees until the cost of $8,000 was paid. The fifth annual session began with 89 students in the new building in 1863.

THE CHICAGO MEDICAL COLLEGE

In the spring of 1863 the Lind University trustees changed the institution's name to Lake Forest University. The medical department then reorganized and adopted a new name, Chicago Medical College. The faculty reorganized, becoming the corporators of the Chicago Medical College and the trustees as well. The Board of Trustees was authorized to fill vacancies on the board, to appoint faculty members, to confer medical degrees on recommendation of the faculty, and to hold legal title to real estate and other property.

NORTHWESTERN UNIVERSITY

Northwestern University was chartered in 1851, eight years before the medical college which would become an affiliate. Both institutions were founded by young professional men of high ideals, courage and dedication to their convictions. They differed in one respect: conformity. The university adhered to established doctrine that religion and learning should follow the patterns of old. It was established under the patronage of the Methodist Episcopal Church, a bond it would share with Wesley Hospital. The medical college, on the other hand, was adventurous in its nonconformity and promotion of a new order of medical education.

In the summer of 1869, when the university's third president, Erastus Otis Haven, took office, he favored medical education and instructed the executive committee to act on "the matter of negotiating with some one of the medical colleges in Chicago with reference to union with the university."

Dr. Nathan S. Davis, who had been a trustee of Northwestern University almost from its inception, reported to the Chicago Medical College faculty "that a union between the two, on just and satisfactory terms, would be desirable." The faculty agreed and negotiations were completed on March 10, 1870.

The agreement was mutually advantageous financially, with the college retaining its corporate name, and control of the faculty and of the curriculum. The university would confer medical degrees and provide $15,000 for a medical building. Northwestern President Haven conferred the medical degrees for the 1869-70 session, thus consummating the union between the university and its new affiliate into the Chicago Medical College, the Medical Department of Northwestern University. A closer union was effected in 1891 and a shorter name, the Northwestern University Medical School, was adopted.

A city ordinance authorized the widening of State Street which would destroy the front of the medical building. The medical college leased a lot adjoining Mercy Hospital and constructed a new building, which was ready for the 12th annual session in 1870-71.

The facilities of another affiliate, St. Luke's Hospital, were added to the annual announcement of Northwestern's medical department for the 1871-72 session. St. Luke's, established in 1864, was located at Indiana Avenue and 16th Street, beyond the reach of the Chicago Fire of 1871. The St. Luke's medical and nursing staffs had been heroic in providing emergency care for the injured during the great disaster.

From 1870 to 1890, the Chicago Medical College of Northwestern University saw its basic principles approved and adopted throughout the country, as the college continued to raise its standards. The original five-month term was increased to seven months by 1889, the year in which a curriculum extending over four years was set up and recommended. The four-year term became obligatory two years later.

By 1890 the college had outgrown its building; enrollment had increased to 237, and space was needed for laboratories and the dispensary. Mercy Hospital not only was unwilling to assign more space to the medical college, but desired the site it already occupied. The Chicago Medical College relinquished its 99-year contract and returned the site to Mercy Hospital.

A Controversial Solution

The spring of 1890 found both Wesley Hospital and the Chicago Medical College without a home. Remembering William Deering's lifelong love of medicine and his support of all interests of the Methodist Episcopal

Church, it could be expected that he would lend a hand to the situation. Deering was a trustee of Northwestern University, of Wesley Hospital, and of the Chicago Training School which sponsored the deaconesses who gave free nursing service to Wesley patients. Deering was further involved as a close friend of Dr. Davis, also a faithful Methodist member who, as dean of Northwestern's medical college, kept Deering informed of its advancements and needs.

According to the Danforth memoirs, the Wesley Executive Committee met informally on April 8, 1890 and "after much discussion, agreed to unite with the Chicago Medical College in securing proposed property at 25th and Dearborn streets as a joint location for the medical college, the hospital, and some other departments of the Northwestern University."

The matter was considered closed because the trustees usually adopted the recommendations of the executive committee, but not this time. There were many harsh words, hurt feelings and disappointments as reflected in these gleanings from Dr. Danforth's notes: "...the best friends of the Chicago Training School for Home and Foreign Missions were particularly anxious that the Hospital should stay on the north side in proximity to the school itself... As the Deaconesses were expected to do the nursing without pay, they at least had reason to expect their wishes to receive consideration... The Reverend Meyer (superintendent) stated that the Deaconess nurses could not serve if the Hospital was moved to the 25th and Dearborn site.

"...On the other hand, the Chicago Medical College, now part of Northwestern University, was equally anxious to have the hospital convenient to Mercy and St. Luke's hospitals which were the chief sources of 'clinical material.' Bedside teaching had become increasingly important in medical schools... Mr. William Deering was and is a firm and generous friend of the University having already given it hundreds of thousands of dollars... It may be assumed that Mr. Deering and Dr. Davis held consultations... and that 'medical college' influence was the main factor which decided where Wesley Hospital would be located, and which influenced Mr. Deering in his purchases of the present location of both college and hospital."

Dr. Danforth continued, "I well remember that Dr. Lucy Rider Meyer went to Evanston to consult with Mr. Deering about reconsidering his decision...I have quite a vivid recollection of her relating the experience. She found Mr. Deering in no very amiable mood, in fact, if I recollect aright, Mr. Deering said 'Take that location or nothing,' although it may have been some other person to whom he used that decisive expression."

Dr. Danforth, of course, understood both sides of the controversy. In the light of medical science and social needs, it was known, even then, that a hospital affiliated with a medical school could give better care to more people and assure future health care. But he also had empathy for the deaconesses, those whose training was primarily religious and whose sole reward was service to mankind. They were apt to view the suffering poor of the present more clearly than the health needs of the future. After all, it had been a mere two generations since deaconesses and sisters, inspired by their clergymen, restored compassionate nursing care to hospitals, then notoriously indifferent to their patients.

WESLEY ACCEPTS NORTHWESTERN SITE

Northwestern University purchased 450 feet of frontage on the east side of Dearborn Street for $41,507, of which William Deering contributed $21,506. The strip extended from 25th Street three-fourths of the way toward 24th Street. The final signing of the contract for land was authorized by the Wesley Board of Trustees at its annual meeting in November, 1890.

The choice corner half of the strip which had 225 feet frontage on Dearborn and 106 feet on 25th Street was sold to Wesley Hospital for $15,340, with deferred payments stipulated in the contract of affiliation (it became a gift in 1899 when the property was deeded to the Hospital for payment of $1.00). It was stipulated that Wesley should erect a hospital whose staff should be drawn from the faculty and that facilities for clinic teaching be afforded the students in the wards and amphitheater of the Hospital. Should these conditions not be met, the title would be returned to Northwestern. The remaining property was assigned to the medical and pharmacy schools.

The Wesley trustees had engaged architects, Treat & Foltz of Chicago, who already were at work. Plans called for three buildings to be erected separately at a total cost of $225,000. However, to meet the urgent need, work began at once on a two-story building that would accommodate about

35 patients and provide administrative space. When larger patient facilities were built, the small building would become a nurses' home.

Hospital Moves to New Building

Patients were moved from the house on East Ohio Street to Wesley's new brick home at 25th and Dearborn streets on November 1, 1891. The Reverend Shelley Meyer, hospital superintendent since its opening, himself had assisted the workmen in completing the desperately needed rooms. Essential furnishings cost $1,000 plus whatever the members of the Ladies Aid Association could muster from their own homes or from friends and neighbors. By December 1, the Hospital was ready for its total capacity of 35 patients, accommodations which would be inadequate all too soon.

On the north end of the 26th Street strip, Northwestern University erected a five-story laboratory building completed in 1893. It contained a large amphitheater, lecture hall and laboratories for research and teaching basic sciences. The four-story Davis Hall, named in honor of the medical school dean, was built between the laboratory building and Wesley Hospital. Davis Hall contained a large and small amphitheater, rooms for the dispensary, library and executive offices.

The impressive university buildings were constructed of brick and cut stone and trimmed with terra cotta, dwarfing the small hospital with its insufficient facilities. For ten years it served under severe handicaps. Patients were carried on stretchers to Davis Hall where their surgery was performed, then returned to the wards the same way. The chance of injury kept physicians and nurses in constant apprehension.

Decade of Contrast   Chapter 5

The decade before the turn of the century marked Chicago's cultural awakening. The symphony orchestra was established in 1890 and affluent citizens purchased paintings in Europe for the new Chicago Art Institute.

For the most part, the developers of great fortunes in Chicago were ambitious, hardworking sons of middle class New Englanders who had applied what little leisure they allowed themselves to health improvement and charitable needs in their adopted city.

CHICAGO HOSTS NATIONS OF THE WORLD

In 1890, Chicago was selected as the site of the World's Columbian Exposition. By an Act of Congress, President Benjamin Harrison had approved an "international exhibit of arts, industries, manufacturers and products of the soil, mines and sea" to which the nations of the world were invited to participate. Harlow N. Higinbotham, who had arranged the first organizational meeting of Wesley Hospital, was named president of the exposition.

Chicago's renowned Louis Sullivan was one of seven architects for the classical buildings of the beautiful white Exposition city on the south shore of Chicago. Parks were planned where 28,000 people could stroll and view the entertainment.

On May 1, 1893, President Grover Cleveland pressed a golden switch which opened the World's Columbian Exposition officially. Chicago Mayor Carter Harrison and Exposition President Harlow Higinbotham hosted European nobility, national dignitaries, Chicago millionaires and persons from every walk of life during the 26 weeks of activities.

So exhilarating and lucrative was the World's Columbian Exposition to Chicago, that the city did not immediately feel the effects of the Panic of 1893, when 15,000 banks and businesses throughout the country went bankrupt. Fear finally overran Chicago on November 1 when families, evicted from their homes, jammed the police stations and City Hall seeking a place to sleep. Children were turned loose in the streets, some finding refuge in the poorhouse.

When a run started on the Illinois Trust and Savings Bank, Philip D. Armour and Marshall Field told anxious depositors who were lined up for their money that all deposits would be personally guaranteed by those two of Chicago's wealthiest men. Harlow Higinbotham had left his closing duties as president of the exposition to assure depositors that their money was safe. When one woman insisted on withdrawing her savings from the bank, Higinbotham held her baby while she waited for the money.[1] Chicago's leaders could not, however, avert the effects of a national depression. Widespread unemployment followed and disease, especially pneumonia, tuberculosis, diptheria and typhoid fever, increased alarmingly.

THE DARKEST HOURS

Despite Wesley Hospital's arrangements with Northwestern University and occupancy of the south side building, the outlook was not bright. The Hospital had begun its third year, 1891, with a deficit of $1,024 which had increased monthly to $1,286 by October 6. In addition, a loan of $8,164 had been obtained from the Metropolitan Bank for the new building. At this time the treasurer, Norman W. Harris, resigned in protest to questionable handling of funds by another officer. A week later, the Reverend J. Shelley Meyer resigned as superintendent (both men were board members and had volunteered their services).

Dr. Danforth wrote, "The early months of 1892 were the darkest hours of Wesley Hospital. It was deeply, almost hopelessly, in debt; its efficient

[1]*Emmett Dedmon, Fabulous Chicago, 1953*

superintendent and treasurer had tendered their resignations, the nursing was unsatisfactory and the Hospital generally was in an unacceptable condition. The operating deficit increased to $1,825 by June and the Reverend George Jeffrey, upon recommendation of Mr. Meyer, was appointed financial agent and superintendent at a salary of $100 per month." This was the first mention of *paid* administration, a subject of dissension among board members.

William H. Rand, president of the board, announced at the annual meeting in November, 1893, the organization of the Wesley Training School for Nurses. The executive committee had endorsed and the board approved a contract to pay six dollars a month to each nurse furnished by the group to Wesley Hospital. This was an abrogation of the contract formerly made with the Chicago Training School. The officers of the Wesley Training School were virtually those of the Deaconess Home; and the nurses, as formerly, were pupils attending the training school.

The former treasurer, Norman W. Harris, volunteered to raise subscriptions sufficient to pay the floating debt, "provided the services of a salaried superintendent were dispensed with," according to Dr. Danforth. The Reverend Joseph Odgers was engaged as superintendent—without salary. High praise was expressed for Anne L. Hewitt, a graduate of St. Luke's Training School, whose proficiency and competence as superintendent of nursing had begun to reverse the inefficiency and slackness that had crept into patient care.

Conditions continued to improve in 1895 when James S. Harvey, a board member, accepted the responsibilities of superintendent and treasurer. Under his direction, debts totaling almost $12,000 were liquidated over the next three years. Repairs for the operating room, plumbing and floors amounting to $634 were made and paid for by small gifts from churches.

In Memory of Mrs. Danforth

A sad occurrence of 1895 was the death of Mrs. Isaac N. Danforth, who founded the Wesley's Ladies Aid Association on March 20, 1889, served as its first president, and worked tirelessly to help meet the needs of the Hospital. Dr. Danforth endowed a patient room, "In loving memory of Elizabeth Skelton Danforth," in Wesley Hospital. Mrs. Danforth also was honored abroad in Kiukiang, Kiangse, China where she had contributed generously to a school sponsored by the Foreign Missions of the Methodist Church. A hospital was built in her memory which is said to still exist.

ENCOURAGING PROSPECTS

In the spring of 1899, Wesley entered into an agreement with the Deaconess Society, turning its management over to the deaconesses for a period of five years. The Hospital was managed through a secondary corporation called the "Wesley Training School Corporation." The Reverend J. Shelley Meyer was welcomed back as superintendent.

The decade ended on an optimistic note when the Board of Trustees, at its annual meeting in November, 1899, named a five-man committee to plan a new building for Wesley Hospital. This committee, comprised of William Deering, Norman W. Harris, James B. Hobbs, Gustavus F. Swift, and the Reverend Robert D. Sheppard who was serving as board president, began its work without delay.

Reaching Maturity
1900 to 1940

Part II

Wesley's New Home   Chapter 6

The year 1900 was more than the start of a new century for Wesley. It was the year that the debt-ridden hospital with 28 beds, 16 pupil nurses, four hired helpers and a $6,000 annual budget, dropped its shackles of poverty. The building committee, named the preceding year, represented some of Chicago's leading industrialists, each of whom gave $500 as a starter and then solicited their colleagues and other businesses for the $237,000 required for a new building. Work started immediately on the brick and steel structure that would accommodate 181 patients. The vacated building would house nurses until 1906, then be used for domestic purposes until 1910, when it would be razed.

Nineteen patients were moved from the "little old building" on June 27, 1901, to attractively furnished rooms in the six-story structure which partially enclosed the old building.

The new part consisted of a center section, a north wing, and an incomplete wing on the south side. In addition to administrative offices, it contained four large wards to accommodate 100 patients, ten smaller wards for 46 patients and 35 private rooms. The surgical facilities consisted of two operating rooms and a clinical amphitheater seating 135 persons. By December, all clinical and patient areas were equipped and decorated.

THE WOMEN'S PART
Even though the Ladies Aid Society treasurer, Mrs. Marcus P. Hatfield,

reported a balance of only twelve cents in the treasury on July 9, 1901, members were not disturbed for they believed they had spent their money well. Through a large bazaar at the Tremont House (Chicago's first hotel on the site of the present Greyhound Bus Terminal at Clark and Lake streets) and other benefits, they had raised $4,263 for furniture, rugs, curtains, linens, silver and china for the new building. Mrs. Sarah E. Wheeler, furnishing committee chairman, was asked to name the men's ward. She promptly called it the "William Deering Ward," in honor of Wesley's chief benefactor.

The Ladies Aid Society meetings had decreased to an average attendance of 23 by 1900, chiefly because of transportation difficulties. Chicago had a new trolley system, an improvement over the former unheated cable cars, but it did not serve all sections of the city. The horse-drawn buggy still was the favorite mode of transportation although more automobiles were appearing on Chicago streets. Only the previous year, Mayor Carter H. Harrison was said to have loudly threatened, "Something must be done about those fellows who run their machines ten to 15 miles an hour!"

Interest engendered by activities concerning the new building increased the women's membership to 157, but meeting attendance continued to be low in 1902. The membership committee, bent on raising attendance, visited one of the "preachers' meetings" held each Monday at the old First Methodist Church at Clark and Washington streets. They asked the ministers to extend invitations to women in their congregations to attend the next meeting of Wesley's Ladies Aid Society. Forty women were present at the following meeting and several new ones joined the society.

A reminder that Chicago winters have been consistent through the years was found in the Ladies Aid minutes of 1905. Recording secretary, Mrs. F.E. Lewis, noted that, "although no regular meetings were held in January or February because of the extremely cold weather, some of our ever-faithful members braved the chilling blasts and storms, going to the meeting room on the regularly appointed days." She added, "If Carnegie does not reward them with a medal, St. Peter will."

INNOVATIONS IN NURSING
The larger hospital required expanded nursing service which brought about changes introduced by Grace Ellsworth, superintendent of nurses and

principal of the training school. Graduate nurses began in 1903 to supervise the student nurses on patient floors and an eight-hour work system was established. The addition of a third year to the course of study improved the program at the Wesley Training School for Nurses. The affiliation with the Northwestern University Medical School made possible a more comprehensive curriculum including laboratory courses in chemistry and bacteriology at the school with classes in anatomy, materia medica, hygiene and nursing given on alternate days. The faculty members, who also were on the Hospital's medical staff, were conscientious, well-prepared lecturers and the extensive medical library was available to the student nurses. It seemed that, almost overnight, Wesley had a top-ranking school of nursing.

The 20 members of the Class of 1903 (sessions had begun before completion of the new building) were addressed by the founder and mentor of Wesley nurses' training, Lucy Rider Meyer, A.M., M.D. The graduate nurses of that year heard Mrs. Meyer, in her inimitable way, trace the history of nursing, which coincided with that of hospitals, from biblical times to her conclusion from which the following is extracted:

"...It is to be remembered with eternal gratitude by the whole civilized world that the entire system of modern trained nurses took its rise directly from this first Deaconess Home and Hospital in Kaiserswerth, Germany[1] (see page xx). For it was to this home that Florence Nightingale[2] went when she would learn nursing. She submitted herself, gentlewoman that she was, to the arduous duties of the sick room. And when, a few years later, a grateful nation poured gold at her feet in recognition of what she had done in the Crimea, she built with the money a great hospital and established in connection with it the *second* Nurses' Training School that was ever in existence; the *first* was at Kaiserswerth. And so there came about our entire modern system of nurses' training schools, and the bright, strong, intelligent, devoted graduate nurse...Whatever the particular

---

[1]*In 1896 Lucy Rider Meyer and her husband, J. Shelley Meyer, made a pilgrimage to the Deaconess Home and Hospital in Kaiserswerth, Germany, where the first deaconesses since those of the early church cared for patients in 1836.*

[2]*In 1905 Mrs. Meyer visited Florence Nightingale in her home in Lea Hurst, England. Miss Nightingale, then an invalid confined to her bed, was alert and pleased to learn of the spread of the deaconess nurse movement in America.*

channel in which your activities flow, remember the sacred origin and glorious history of your profession, and honor it, by earnest and conscientious devotion..."

WESLEY WAS READY

The Hospital was alerted on December 30, 1903, to prepare for an unknown number of persons burned in Chicago's most tragic fire since 1871. The setting was the Iroquois Theater, an ornate showplace with a plush and mahogany lobby. An overflowing matinee audience of 1,600, mostly women and children, saw a flash of flame from an overloaded electrical circuit ignite a drapery at the side of the stage. A blast of fire swept into the auditorium and up toward the balconies and galleries which became an inferno of flames and panic. Victims were piled five and six deep before the locked fire doors and exits, which opened inward.

It was estimated that the fire was out within half an hour, yet counting the dead lasted a day and a night. The coroner said there were 601 bodies, only one of which was unidentified, according to newspaper accounts of the disaster.

Wesley Hospital's records showed that 209 victims with various degrees of burns were brought in over a three-week period from December 30 through January 19, 1904.

DEACONESS MANAGEMENT ENDS

From 1899 through 1904, Wesley had been under the administration of the Methodist Deaconess Society. This period had included Wesley's most difficult time to date when heavy debt precluded proper facilities to care for the constant flow of patients. The deaconesses had valiantly nursed the sick under trying conditions. Their service, without compensation, was a large factor in gaining the strength and support Wesley needed to become a first-class hospital.

The five-year agreement expired at the end of 1904 and it was mutually agreed, in view of the rapid growth and subsequent administrative responsibility, that the Wesley Hospital Corporation reassume management of the property in its own name.

GENERAL STATISTICS

Dr. A. Dudley Jackson, a trustee and medical staff member, was acting superintendent during Wesley's transition from a 28-bed hospital to one accommodating 181 patients. He remained in office until 1908. His report for the year ending December 31, 1904, announced record admissions of 2,785 patients, of whom 1,155 were surgical, 417 gynecological, 589 medical, 280 nose and throat, 122 obstetrical, 115 orthopedic, 50 eye and ear, and 57 pediatric cases. Births numbered 75. The five most common conditions were appendicitis, 207; typhoid fever, 58; inguinal hernia, 53; pneumonia, 36; and rheumatism, 33. There were 170 deaths.

The total cost of maintaining the Hospital for the year 1904 was $80,021.67; the cost per patient day was $1.88. Charity and part pay patients numbered 430 and their care cost the Hospital $9,869.80. Wesley received $6,919.53 in contributions plus $543.80 from endowment funds for maintenance in 1904. The year's deficit was $4,138.

The diversity of people served by Wesley was shown in a table in the Annual Report classifying patients' nationalities. More than two thirds were Americans; 696 patients were foreign born and not yet United States citizens. A total of 550 patients were from eight countries: Germany, 261; Ireland, 97; Sweden, 76; Greece, 32; England, 28; Canada, 26; France, 15, and Poland, 15. The remaining 146 patients were from 11 other countries including Bohemia, China, Denmark, Holland, Hungary, Italy, Norway, Russia, Spain, Turkey and Wales. Within its 16 years of existence, Wesley had become international in its patient population.

Lifelong Friends of Wesley   Chapter 7

The election of Perley Lowe, a Wesley trustee since 1894, as president of the board in 1904 began an important section in the hospital's annals. He succeeded Robert D. Sheppard, D.D., who had become president in 1892.

Mr. Lowe was a lumberman from Levant, Maine, who had moved his family to Chicago in 1867. He established a successful lumber company in his adopted city and served several terms as a director, vice president and president of the Illinois Lumberman's Exchange. He was an active member of the Methodist Church, a delegate from the Rock River Conference to the General Methodist Conference in Los Angeles, and a trustee of Northwestern University.

One of the first duties accepted by Lowe as a Wesley trustee was that of auditor, a service previously performed by unpaid workers, some of whom were not adept at bookkeeping. The small anomalies which had been adjusted in a 28-bed hospital, were not acceptable in a large one with greater financial responsibility. As auditor, Mr. Lowe worked closely with Dr. A. Dudley Jackson, Wesley superintendent and professor of materia medica and anatomy at Northwestern's medical school and the Hospital's school of nursing. It soon became apparent to both men that a destructive element was undermining the institution.

The episode was described in the book, *The Methodist Movement in Northern Illinois* by Almer M. Pennewell, president of the Rock River

Conference Historical Society. In his chapter on Wesley's origin, he wrote "At this time (1903), working hand-in-glove with Dr. Jackson, was Mr. Perley Lowe. As eager as the superintendent to diagnose the case, Lowe set his keen, analytical business mind to work, and, using the business man's knowledge that trust is more often betrayed than any other virtue, ran the quarry down..." It was revealed that a respected citizen had been using the Hospital for his own gain, but the person was not named.

Commenting on Perley Lowe's 20-year presidential tenure, Dr. Pennewell wrote: "No pen could enumerate the sacrifices Mr. Lowe made from this period until the day of his death, July 29, 1924, to keep Wesley Hospital out of financial and managerial difficulties."

THE HARRIS HOME FOR NURSES

An urgently needed addition to Wesley in the spring of 1906 was the Harris Home for Nurses, erected on South Dearborn Street, one block north of the Hospital. The $30,000 residence was the gift of Norman Wait Harris, president of the Harris Trust & Savings Bank of Chicago. Before joining the Wesley board in 1888, he was president of the board of the Chicago Training School for Home and Foreign Missions (Wesley Hospital's birthplace), and of the Deaconess Pension Fund which he founded and to which he donated $100,000. He also was on the board of Northwestern University, to which he gave $250,000 to erect the Harris Hall of Political Science and History. Of his five children, two would remain in Chicago and continue their father's interest in Wesley. They were Norman Dwight Harris who was elected to the board in 1937, and Pearl Emma Harris who, in 1910, was married to M. Hadden MacLean who became a Wesley trustee in 1918.

The Harris Home for Nurses was a morale builder for 80 Wesley nurses who had been packed into the structure designed for 30 patients back in 1899. It also was an incentive to the Ladies Aid members who borrowed $5,000 to furnish the new home, their note guaranteed by the board president, Perley Lowe. Activities accelerated to the extent that many women waived their customary summer vacations to shop for furnishings for the new home and to persuade friends to donate special equipment. On the evening of September 25, 1906, with draperies hung, furniture placed and complimentary flowers arranged, the women were hostesses at the opening of the Harris Home for Nurses. As carriage after carriage of friends arrived, "the sound of horses' hooves was accented by the occasional backfire of a balky automobile," according to the vivid minutes of the Ladies Aid Society.

THE BAZAAR OF NATIONS

A year and a month passed before the loan to the Ladies Aid Society was retired, so elaborate were plans to raise the money. But when preparations took shape for "The Bazaar of Nations," Chicagoans knew it would be an extraordinary affair.

The Bazaar of Nations was named by its chairman, Mrs. (Marion Martin) George William Dixon, daughter-in-law of the influential Arthur Dixons, and a new member of the Ladies Aid Society. Her committee included Mrs. Norman Wait Harris, treasurer; Mrs. James Frake, recording secretary; Mrs. James B. Gascoigne, corresponding secretary; and 35 vice presidents.

The widely publicized Bazaar of Nations opened Thursday evening, November 7, 1907, and continued through November 9. The old First Regiment Armory at 15th Street and South Michigan Avenue had been transformed into a miniature antecedent of the United Nations. Twenty booths were structured in the characteristic architecture of the nations represented which included America, Belgium, China, Egypt, England, France, Germany, Greece, Holland, Hungary, India, Ireland, Italy, Japan, Norway, Palestine, Persia, Russia, Spain and Switzerland. Women attending the booths wore the native dress of the country represented, the American attire being of the colonial period. A model hospital was exhibited and music was provided by the First Regiment Armory band.

Illinois Governor Charles S. Deneen gave the opening address and Chicago Mayor Fred A. Busse presented Mrs. Dixon with a small gold key, the "key to the situation," he called it, which she wore on a chain around her neck. The bazaar netted $11,000, which enabled the women to pay their loan, install a passenger elevator in the Hospital, provide food warmers and a refrigeration system for the kitchen.

THE DIXONS

Arthur Dixon and his wife, Annie Carson Dixon, had made substantial contributions to Wesley, to other institutions sponsored by the Methodist

Church, and to Chicago philanthropy in general. Born in Ireland, Dixon was president of the Irish-Republican Club of Chicago, was active in enlisting and equipping men for service in the Civil War, and was a delegate to the National Republican Convention in 1880. He founded and was president of the Arthur Dixon Transfer Company and a large stockholder in several businesses. Mr. Dixon served as a member of the Wesley Board of Trustees from 1899 until his death in 1917. Of the Dixons' 14 sons and daughters, several followed their parents' philanthropic precedent, which continued for several generations.

A sequel of the Dixon legend is contained in a manuscript entitled *Fruit of Their Years, a History of the Woman's Auxiliary of Chicago Wesley Memorial Hospital, March 20, 1889—May 31, 1957* by Mrs. J. Bert (Mae S.) Wilson, a member who served as treasurer. The incident concerns the group's 1903 president, a hospital trustee, Mrs. George (Sarah E.) Wheeler, known as "Aunt Sarah" at Wesley where she volunteered countless service hours until her death in 1923 at the age of 82.

Aunt Sarah was disturbed because of perenially poor attendance at Ladies Aid meetings. Mrs. Wilson's account of Aunt Sarah's solution follows:

> One day she (Aunt Sarah) had an inspiration. As her motto for over forty years had been, "Now then, do it!" (see page 15 for origin of motto), she immediately put on her wraps and went down to the Arthur Dixon Transfer Company at 299 Fifth Avenue, now called South Wells Street, picking her way between the drays and horses, to Mr. Dixon's office.
>
> "Arthur," she said, punctuating her remarks with thumpings of her cane, "You have a houseful of women. We want one of them for president of our Ladies Aid of Wesley."
>
> "All right," he replied.
>
> Turning to his son, Aunt Sarah continued, "George, what is the matter with your wife being our new president?"
>
> "Aunt Sarah, if you elect her, I'll see that she gets there," George Dixon promised.
>
> Shortly after, a committee called on Mrs. George Dixon to ask if she would serve as president. Before accepting, Mrs. Dixon asked why the group thought she would be a better president than others who had been members for a longer time. She also asked a number of questions dealing with the scope of the work, future aims of the Ladies Aid Society and the responsibilities of the office of president. Only after receiving satisfactory answers to all of these questions, did she accept.

Mrs. George W. Dixon was to serve as president of the Wesley Ladies Aid Society from 1908 until her death in 1926. Her husband was president of the Board of Trustees (1924 to 1934) for 10 of his 24 years on the board. Their son, George W. Dixon, Jr., was a Wesley trustee from 1941 until his death in 1966, and vice president of the Board from 1942 to 1951.

Two other sons of Arthur and Annie Dixon, William W. and Homer L., and a grandson, Wesley Moon Dixon, gave long and honorable service to the Hospital. These descendants and others[1] are interwoven in the history of Wesley Hospital.

ADMINISTRATIVE APPOINTMENTS

In April, 1908, Eugene S. Gilmore, formerly associated with the University of Michigan Hospital at Ann Arbor, Michigan, succeeded Dr. Jackson as superintendent of Wesley. During his 23 years as the Hospital's chief executive officer, Gilmore served as a trustee and president (1925) of the American Hospital Association; vice president of the Protestant Hospital Association; secretary and trustee of the Methodist Hospitals & Homes Association; and general consultant for architects, superintendents and others interested in planning new hospitals. The qualifications necessary to fill these offices would serve Wesley well, especially during the next two years (1908-1910) when the south wing would be completed.

Another administrative appointment was made in September when Bertha L. Knapp, graduate of the University Hospital at Ann Arbor, joined Wesley as superintendent of nurses and director of the school of nursing.

Anticipating the need for more nurses in the south wing, Wesley purchased, for $7,000, the property of the Chicago Charity Hospital just north of Northwestern's medical school early in 1910. The land, with 25 feet of frontage on Dearborn Street, had a three-story brick building which would be used as an annex of the Harris Home to lodge first year student nurses. This was the first of several holdings Wesley would acquire from institutions terminating their service. Interns occupied a three-story house on State Street valued at $160,000, a Deering donation.

[1]*After Wesley and Passavant hospitals merged in 1972, Mrs. (Suzanne Searle) Wesley Moon Dixon, wife of a great grandson of the Arthur Dixons, became president of the Woman's Board of Northwestern Memorial Hospital (Wesley-Passavant united), 1976.*

Dr. Danforth's Tribute to Dr. Davis

After the death of Dr. Nathan Smith Davis in June, 1904, Dr. Danforth had continued the formidable task he already had begun, writing the Davis biography. Although, in 1889, Dr. Danforth and Dr. Davis had differed in their opinions of the best location for Wesley, these two men of high purpose became fast friends as colleagues on the faculty of Northwestern Medical School.

The well-documented book, *The Life of Nathan Smith Davis, A.M., M.D., LL.D. 1817-1904,* by I.N. Danforth, A.M., M.D., was published by the Cleveland Press, Chicago, Illinois, in 1907. It delineated Davis's youth and medical studies, professional life and association with the Chicago Medical College and other educational and charitable institutions; his work with the American Medical Association and other professional organizations; his religious and church life, temperance work, character and personality. The book is a scholarly portrayal of a great man's accomplishments in health and medicine, presented with the warm understanding of a fellow physician. In the preface, dated September, 1907, Dr. Danforth stated:

"I began writing the life of Dr. Davis with great reluctance; I close with greater reluctance. For several months past he has been my constant companion. I might almost say, day and night. As I have studied his austere personality, and his rugged character, so transparent and genuine, my respect for the man has grown day by day. A character so colossal needs the perspective of time and distance, before an adequate estimate of its merits or demerits can be formed.

"Just at this point, the mail brings me the following letter from the present Dr. N.S. Davis, worthy successor of a noble father, which it gives me great pleasure to receive and print:

My dear Doctor Danforth:

You have striven most conscientiously to present correctly the facts in my father's life and I believe that you have succeeded.

Unfortunately there have been few manuscript aids for the construction of your work, and my father's contemporaries are almost all dead. However, in spite of these difficulties you have successfully described the important incidents of his life.

It has been a pleasure to aid you as far as possible.

Very sincerely yours,
N. S. Davis

Dr. Danforth had resumed work on his Wesley memoirs in July, 1910 when he wrote:

"On the morning of December 11, 1909, my friend, Dr. Marcus P. Hatfield, died at Wesley Hospital after a long and distressing illness. During his several months in the hospital, every nurse, intern and all who were connected with the hospital were unwearied in their constant, tender care...I first knew Mark Hatfield as a lively fellow of 18, open-hearted, frank with a somewhat fiery temper...then as a student in the Chicago Medical College whence he graduated in 1872...a few years later we were colleagues on the faculty of the Nothwestern Medical School...later still, we were most intimately associated in the work of setting Wesley Hospital on its legs and helping to tide it over its callow days...During his long and faithful service to Wesley Hospital, Dr. Hatfield was a trustee, secretary of the Executive Committee, secretary of the Medical Board, and an unremittingly faithful physician to the Children's Department..."

The remainder of Dr. Danforth's memoirs are incorporated in earlier pages. The founder of Wesley had the pleasure of seeing his son, William Clark Danforth, graduate from Northwestern University Medical School in 1903. After taking postgraduate work in Vienna, the young Dr. Danforth returned to the states and was married to Miss Gertrude MacLean of New York. He practiced first in Chicago, then at Evanston Hospital where he became chief of the department of obstetrics and gynecology.

The W. C. Danforths had a son, David Newton Danforth, who, like his father, was graduated from Northwestern University Medical School. He began his practice at Wesley, and shortly thereafter became chief of obstetrics and gynecology at Evanston Hospital. He returned to Wesley in 1965 as chairman of obstetrics and gynecology and chairman of the department at Northwestern, where he remained until 1972. The three generations of Danforth physicians served on the faculty of Northwestern University Medical School.

Medical World Mourns Death of Wesley's Founder

The sad announcement of Dr. Isaac Newton Danforth's death on May 5, 1911, at the age of 76 brought condolences to his family and friends at Wesley from throughout the medical world. Dr. Danforth had retired from active practice in 1895 because of illness, but continued his professional appointments for two years. He had nurtured the small Wesley Hospital in the mission training school to which he had sent its first patient on Christmas day, 1888, had organized its board and medical staff, and watched it mature for 22 years.

Wesley 1910: Enlarged and Modern　　Chapter 8

esley's six-story south wing was opened Saturday, May 7, 1910, with 54 beds, increasing the patient complement to 225. This placed Wesley, in its twenty-first year, among the largest and most modern hospitals in Chicago. Governor Charles S. Deneen again was on hand to address the group along with Judge Oliver H. Horton. Their wives, both officers of the Ladies Aid Society, were in the receiving line headed by Mrs. George W. Dixon.

Nearly a thousand friends toured the new wing viewing the clinical amphitheater, the X-ray unit, hydrotherapy room and—most remarkable for that time—the surgical suite. The guide explained that 20 rooms were devoted directly to surgery: rooms for operating, for preparing patients, for doctors and nurses to scrub, for sterilizing and keeping instruments, bandages and general supplies. In 1910, scarcely 40 years since the vile era of "laudable pus," this was the complete antithesis—momentous to those who remembered the terrifying years.

Guests were guided through the wards where air was regulated to meet the needs of contagious cases, and through mahogany-furnished private rooms. On the roof was a glass-enclosed sun parlor and a veranda with a gazebo, rustic seat and swinging hammock. Here patients could view Lake Michigan as they convalesced in comfort.

Deering Emphasizes Wesley's Purposes

The new wing had been constructed at a cost of $137,000, of which William Deering had donated $55,000 and Mrs. Deering, $20,000. The entire Wesley plant, exclusive of Northwestern's medical school which was adjacent to the Hospital and an essential part of its assets, was valued at approximately half a million dollars. In addition, at the beginning of 1911 there was an accumulated endowment fund of $269,043.47, of which Mr. Deering had given $225,000.

In 1901 William Deering had decided to retire a second time from business and to devote his special aptitudes of good judgment, recognition of advantageous opportunities and prompt application of energy—factors that had gained him two fortunes—to his philanthropic interests. At 75, he was in fine physical condition to enjoy extended winters, November through May, at Coconut Grove, Florida, about five miles south of Miami, where the Deerings had a cottage and a few acres of land facing Biscayne Bay. In friendly letters to Wesley colleagues Perley Lowe, president, and Norman W. Harris, treasurer, he extolled the soft breezes and blue waters, urging them to take winter vacations in the Biscayne area which "has the most equitable and mildest climate in America." His letters were filled with kindly sympathy for their disappointments when efforts failed, with suggestions and solicitous words of encouragement as well as astute advice.

There was one point where Mr. Deering was adamant: that Wesley Hospital and Northwestern University Medical School cooperate according to the terms of affiliation. In 1906 rumors of differences between the hospital and medical school had come to Mr. Deering's attention. He wrote to Norman Harris, with whom he had discussed the matter, emphasizing "that the hospital was established on a basis that would be satisfactory and obtain the support first, of all the Methodist people; second, of the friends and supporters of the Deaconess' work; and third, supply an absolute necessity to an excellent medical school."

In 1907, Deering explained his point more clearly. In reply to Perley Lowe's reminder of another building fund started by trustees, Mr. Deering wrote that he had delayed stating his subscription for two reasons: "I want a complete and full understanding and agreement between the two benefic-iaries for which Wesley Hospital was originally started and founded: viz., the Hospital itself for hospital purposes, and to benefit and assist the

Northwestern University Medical School. These were the two objects for which it was founded and no one then connected with it, misunderstood the matter." Deering implied that the latecomers who wished to modify and divert the founding purposes, would understand the original agreement, if properly presented, and carry it out in good faith. Until there was practical unanimity with the friends and trustees of the hospital and medical school, Mr. Deering declined to name his subscription.

Adjustments were made, at least temporarily, and William Deering contributed liberally to the south wing. In March, 1911, Perley Lowe wrote Deering that a $100,000 long-standing Wesley debt was finally paid. Deering responded, "You have done one of the best and most successful jobs of a good and charitable life work and I thank and congratulate you." This communication of April 9, 1911, was the last one in the Wesley records to Perley Lowe from his great friend and counselor, William Deering.

Charles, the elder Deering son, and his half brother, James, spent much of 1912 and 1913 with their father, whose health was failing. Their sister, Abby Deering Howe, had died in 1906. James had visited Wesley while in Chicago and was conducted on a comprehensive tour by Eugene S. Gilmore, superintendent. The Deering sons gradually assumed their father's philanthropic interests and continued the Wesley correspondence.

The Supreme Gift: Health for the Multitude

After a brief illness, death came quietly to William Deering on the evening of Tuesday, December 9, 1913, in his 87th year. His wife and two sons, James and Charles; and his attending physician, Dr. P.T. Skaggs, were at his bedside in the modest cottage at Coconut Grove. His body, accompanied by his family, was carried by train to Evanston, Illinois, for burial.

Of the thousands of tributes paid to William Deering from throughout the world, perhaps the most appropriate to Wesley's history was given by Bishop William Fraser McDowell at the funeral services in the First Methodist Episcopal Church in Evanston, where William Deering worshipped during the most productive part of his remarkable life.

In part, Bishop McDowell spoke of William Deering in these words: "In view of what he has actually achieved in the line of life he followed, it is rather interesting to know that more than once in these later years he referred tenderly, almost wistfully and longingly, to an early ambition to be a country doctor. He began the study of medicine in his youth and was obliged to give it up... And once at least he was heard to express the hope that in character and ministry to human life he might have been such a physician as his dear friend, the late Nathan Davis. He saw in that noble man and great physician what he liked to think he himself might have been...

"He might have been a country doctor of the old school, leaving behind him at last the single practioner's list of grateful and happy patients. He thought it a strange providence, rather a hard providence, that kept him from that career...

"Through Wesley Hospital, and in related ways, he has done those vastly greater things by bringing the skill and service of the many to the need of the ailing multitude. He has been more a physician, after all, than even in his largest young dream he ever fancied he might be. And this is one of God's good ways of bringing compensations to men."

Bickering Beneficiaries

Wesley's Annual Reports after 1909 had shown vastly improved facilities and greater service each year, but the discord between the hospital and medical school had not abated. Correspondence between the Deering brothers and hospital executives indicated that the sons were conscientiously continuing their father's humanitarian interests.

Charles Deering, acting on a suggestion of Perley Lowe in 1911, had purchased property at the north end of State Street which he intended to give to Wesley. On May 22, 1913, Lowe wrote to Charles who was visiting Paris, describing the core of the friction between Wesley Hospital and the medical school. He pointed out that when the property on which it then stood was deeded to Wesley, it was upon the express condition that "the staff of the Hospital be drawn from the faculties of Northwestern University Medical School and facilities for clinic teaching be afforded students of the school in the wards and amphitheatre of the hospital, as required by the grantor herein." On failure of Wesley Hospital to carry out these conditions, the title would revert to Northwestern University, according to the Deed of Conveyance.

Lowe claimed that the above was later supplemented by a contract stating that the staff should be *nominated* by the university and *confirmed* by the hospital trustees. Wesley trustees had often thought it advantageous to add other physicians, but the university, having the power to veto or refuse to confirm their nominations, would not consent.

Lowe continued, "There has been no serious trouble until this year when the hospital refused to accept a few men whom we considered undesirable, from the hospital viewpoint. The university also claims the right to assign the doctors to the place on our staff they wish them to occupy. This, we claim, should be the right of the hospital. The practical outworking is that it is within Northwestern's power to nominate a staff too small for the proper operation of the hospital and, also, to prevent us from getting the best talent available outside its faculty. In addition, the university may nominate any person for a particular place on our staff, and we must go without anyone for that place, unless we are willing to accept the one they wish..."

Perley Lowe then proposed a solution: "Now, if you are willing to deed us this property, I suggest that you write a letter to Northwestern University...saying that, at your request, I had sent- you a copy of the Deed of Conveyance and advised you of the existing conditions and that if Northwestern would cancel its claims upon Wesley, you would then deed the hospital the balance of the State Street property."

Charges of the university against the hospital had reached the Deerings even before William Deering's health had declined. The school had claimed that its students were not admitted to the wards and that eminent faculty members, properly recommended, had been excluded from the hospital staff.

Undoubtedly the Deering sons shielded their invalid father from the festering dissension between his two beloved benevolences, and no action was taken in 1913.

Wesley Commemorates Its Benefactors

Chapter 9

James Deering began the year, 1914, with a request on January 2 to Wesley Hospital for its current Annual Report. He was sent the review of its twenty-fifth year, which ended December 31, 1913, on an active, prosperous note. In a quarter of a century, the Hospital had grown from four meagerly furnished rooms to a 225-bed institution, free of debt with total resources amounting to $1,899,306.83. The income for the year was $188,927.33 and expenses were $169,918.46, leaving a balance of $19,008.87. This was applied to a deficit of $15,430.08 for free care, leaving a net surplus of $3,578.79. Donations from Methodist churches totaled $21,334.39.

Patients admitted during 1913 numbered 5,342 with an average stay of 12 days at a per diem cost of $3.08. Twenty-eight percent were free or part pay patients. Wesley was said to lead all voluntary Chicago hospitals in the percentage of free care given. Sixty charity beds were maintained for adults and four-fifths of the work in the children's ward was free. The number of operations performed was 3,562, placing Wesley ahead of other Chicago hospitals in the amount of surgical work done.

Listed in the Annual Report were the officers and 29 members of the Board of Trustees:

H.O. Tomlinson, Owner, publisher and book brokerage firm
Edwin L. Wagner, President, National Produce Bank; Berwyn State Bank
The Medical Staff was composed of 64 physicians with status of emeritus, attending, adjunct or assisting. Fifteen Northwestern graduates served two-year internships.

MEDICAL STAFF
William E. Schroeder, M.D., Chief of Staff
Frederick Menge, M.D., Secretary

MEDICINE
Emeritus:
Robert Preble, M.D.
Nathan S. Davis, M.D.
Attending:
Charles A. Elliott, M.D.
Achilles Davis, M.D.
Luther J. Osgood, M.D.
Alexander A. Goldsmith, M.D.
James F. Churchill, M.D.
Adjunct:
George G. Dwan, M.D.
Arthur Beifeld, M.D.
Thomas P. Foley, M.D.
James G. Carr, M.D.
Assistant:
John W. Miller, M.D.
Walter H. Buehlig, M.D.
George D.J. Griffin, M.D.
John M. Lilly, M.D.
Hugo W. Traub, M.D.

SURGERY
Attending:
William E. Schroeder, M.D.
Frederick A. Besley, M.D.
Harry M. Richter, M.D.
Allen B. Kanavel, M.D.
Adjunct:
William R. Cubbins, M.D.
Charles M. Fox, M.D.

John A. Wolfer, M.D.
Paul B. Magnuson, M.D.
Assistant:
William E. Shackleton, M.D.
Arthur L. Shreffler, M.D.
Jacob R. Buchbinder, M.D.
Lester H. Hills, M.D.

PATHOLOGY
Attending:
Frederick R. Zeit, M.D.
William H. Holmes, M.D.

NOSE AND THROAT
Attending:
Frederick Menge, M.D.
Adjunct:
Charles B. Younger, M.D.
George J. Dennis, M.D.
Otis H. McClay, M.D.
Assistant:
E.S. Stewart, M.D.

OPHTHALMOLOGY
Attending:
Brown Pusey, M.D.

BACTERIOLOGY
Attending:
Arthur I. Kendall, M.D.

GYNECOLOGY
Attending:
Mark T. Goldstine, M.D.
Robert T. Gillmore, M.D.
Assistant:
O.S. Pavlik, M.D.
Payson L. Nusbaum, M.D.
Christian D. Hauch, M.D.

OBSTETRICS
Attending:
Charles B. Reed, M.D.
Adjunct:
Herbert M. Stowe, M.D.
David S. Hillis, M.D.

DERMATOLOGY
Attending:
Joseph Zeisler, M.D.
Frank E. Simpson, M.D.

PEDIATRICS
Attending:
Joseph Brenneman, M.D.
Robert A. Krost, M.D.
Assistant:
F.B. Combs, M.D.

NEUROLOGY
Emeritus:
Archibald Church, M.D.
Hugh T. Patrick, M.D.
Attending:
D'Orsay Hecht, M.D.
Julius Grinker, M.D.
Assistant:
Albert B. Yudelson, M.D.
Adjunct:
George T. Jordan, M.D.
Robert Blue, M.D.

OTOLOGY
Attending:
J. Gordon Wilson, M.D.
Assistant:
Walter T. McGibbon, M.D.
Lawrence E. Sleeper, M.D.
Carl F. Bookwalter, M.D.

GENITO URINARY
Attending:
Louis E. Schmidt, M.D.
Adjunct:
V.D. Lespinasse, M.D.

RESEARCH PROJECTS FOR INTERNS

A medical innovation at Wesley was the establishment of five research fellowships for interns who had completed their service and desired to conduct studies directed by attending physicians. The projects were (1) phlyctenular conjunctivitis, a recurring inflammation of the eye which occurred frequently in children and could result in serious injury to vision, directed by Dr. Brown Pusey, Northwestern chairman of ophthalmology, and Dr. Joseph Brenneman, pediatrician; (2) tuberculin, its preparation and potency as a possible cure for tuberculosis, supervised by Dr. Arthur I. Kendall, Northwestern chairman of bacteriology; (3) comparing figures from examinations of urine from diseased kidneys with that of normal cases to determine change and basis for treatment, directed by Dr. Charles A. Elliott, Northwestern chairman of medicine (1917-1937); (4) action of the liver and kidneys during and following anesthetic to develop means of alleviating injurious effects of anesthesia and prevent complication, directed by Dr. Allen B. Kanavel, chairman of surgery (1919-1929); (5) studying infant feeding to determine the predominating intestinal bacteria in various diets and how changes could be brought about by correcting the diets, directed by Drs. Kendall and Brenneman.

THE DEERING GIFT

Judging by the facts and figures sent to James Deering at the beginning of 1914, Wesley was an outstanding hospital with a progressive program of patient care, medical education, research, and affiliation with a leading university. The Board of Trustees represented the sound responsibility to be expected from religious, civic and business leaders. The financial statement reflected careful management and the statistical report of service given indicated an institution that was vital to the city's health. The distinction of the medical staff could not be refuted. The fact that four current or future chairmen of Northwestern University medical departments participated in Wesley's five new research projects unquestionably denoted cooperation between the medical school and hospital (though not as much as the school had demanded).

By 1914, Wesley had become the institution that William Deering had so wanted it to be—a teaching hospital providing health care to the poor and wealthy alike, offering clinical facilities and experience to medical students, while receiving strong support from the Methodist Church.

It was to be expected that James Deering would select Wesley Hospital as the appropriate memorial to his father, William Deering, and sister, Abby Deering Howe. Accordingly, the Deed of Gift, notarized April 9, 1914, of more than one million dollars to Wesley Hospital was received, accepted and announced to the public.

A certified copy of the Deed of Gift which stipulated that the name, Wesley Hospital, be changed to Wesley Memorial Hospital to commemorate the donor's father and sister, is printed here in its entirety.

KNOW ALL MEN BY THESE PRESENTS, That I, James Deering of the city and state of New York, do hereby give and grant to the WESLEY HOSPITAL, a corporation organized and existing under the laws of the state of Illinois, now maintaining a hospital in the city of Chicago, the municipal bonds listed on the schedule hereto attached. In the month of December, 1913, a valuation was placed on these bonds by the First Trust and Savings Bank of Chicago, of Nine hundred eighty-five thousand, nine hundred sixty-five and 25/100 Dollars ($985,965.25), which, with the accumulated interest, makes a total value of One million, two hundred thirteen and 08/100 Dollars ($1,000,213.08), as is shown in and by the aforesaid schedule.

The Wesley Hospital is to have and to hold said fund unto it and its successors, in perpetual trust, for the charitable use herein specified, and upon the conditions following; namely:

(1) The corporate name of the Wesley Hospital shall be changed to Wesley Memorial Hospital. A tablet of appropriate size shall be placed and maintained in the Hospital explaining that the word "Memorial" in the name aforesaid is used to signify that the Hospital is a memorial to William Deering and Abby Deering Howe. In the annual reports and other publications published by the Hospital, and on the letterheads and stationery used therein the same fact shall appear in an appropriate way.

(2) It is my purpose that the fund hereby created shall be devoted to the charity work of the Hospital. The fund itself shall not be used, but only the income therefrom is to be used for the purposes specified. I am willing that from any accumulation of interest from this fund, buildings shall be erected for charity patients, or fixtures or appliances needed in the hospital for charity work, may be purchased. The charity work provided for under this endowment shall be so conducted as to contribute everything to real charity

but nothing to mendicancy or pauperism. To this end, I direct that the Hospital shall put itself in sympathetic connection with organized charities in Chicago, and especially with such organizations as investigate the operations, character and work of other charities. I direct that by the Hospital's own paid or volunteer workers, or in cooperation with the Visiting Nurse Association of Chicago, or other like agencies, a thorough investigation be made as to the merits of all charity patients accepted under this bequest, and a record of such investigation shall be kept for the use of the Hospital and for the use of any other charitable institution or organization in the city of Chicago that desires the same.

I further direct that through the agencies and by the methods last aforesaid, or otherwise, cases of misfortune and misery may be sought out and relieved as far as possible. I direct that such out-service maternity and other cases be given as the Trustees of the Hospital may deem wise and expedient.

To the extent that the Trustees of the Hospital deem it wise, I shall be glad to have public lectures on hygiene and the prevention and cure of disease given the poor, either in the hospital or elsewhere.

(3) It is my belief that the best hospital is the one that has close relations with a good medical school, and the best medical school is the one that has close relations with a complete and well-conducted hospital. For this reason, I desire the Medical School of Northwestern University and Wesley Memorial Hospital to act in close and friendly relation with each other. To this end, I specify that the President of Northwestern University, the Dean of its Medical Department, and an additional member of its Board of Trustees, selected by its Executive Committee, all of whom shall also be members of such Executive Committee, shall always be members of the Board of Trustees of Wesley Memorial Hospital. The additional member above specified to be one who can and will be active and attentive to the affairs of the University and the Hospital. The duties and powers of the aforesaid Dean, as a member of such Executive Committee, may be restricted to the relations between the University and the Hospital. The three persons so specified also to be constituted, by a resolution or by-law adopted by the Board of Trustees of the University, a committee on relations between the University and the Hospital.

Also, the President of Wesley Memorial Hospital, its Superintendent, and an additional member of its Board of Trustees, selected by the Executive Committee, all of whom shall also be members of such Executive Committee, shall also be members of the Board of Trustees of Northwestern University. The additional member, above specified, to be one who can and will be active and attentive to the affairs of the University and the Hospital.

The three persons aforesaid to be constituted, by a resolution or by-law adopted by the Board of Trustees of the Hospital, a committee on relations between the Hospital and the University. These two committees so selected from the University and the Hospital respectively, as aforesaid, shall meet together at least once each month for the discussion and consideration of the joint interests of the Hospital and University, and the committee may decide all questions that arise in so far as they are severally authorized so to do by their respective Boards of Trustees. If any member habitually neglects the meetings of said committee, or is otherwise neglectful of the affairs of the University or Hospital, he shall be removed from the Committee by the Executive Committee appointing him, and his place shall be supplied by another appointment.

(4) Under this gift, Wesley Memorial Hospital shall be a teaching hospital and, both in the charity work herein provided for, and everywhere else in the hospital, it shall give all proper teaching facilities consistent with the principle that the patient's welfare is the first consideration. The Medical Department must maintain and strictly enforce a high standard of preparatory studies for the admission of students. The Medical School must provide an adequate staff for the Hospital.

It is my hope that the time will come when, by mutual agreement between the School and the Hospital, an appointment to the faculty of the school will be an *ipso facto* appointment to the staff of the Hospital, but I do not now insist upon this.

I recognize that in a medical school and hospital united in work and sympathy and united physically, the matter of a free dispensary and laboratories are of mutual interest. I am willing that a portion of the income from this endowment, bearing the same relation to the total income of the Medical School and the Hospital, shall be expended for the operation and conduct of such dispensary and laboratories; the School and the Hospital contributing to the expense on the same basis.

(5) Realizing that many functions of the Hospital must be used in common for the good both of the charity patients herein provided for and the other patients, I direct that for such functions as are clearly of this character such a proportion of the income of the fund herein provided a shall cause the charity work herein provided for to bear its fair share of the cost with the other work of the Hospital shall be so expended. But for the purposes of this deed of gift, the Hospital, in computing its expenditures in charity cases, shall proceed as follows: It shall ascertain and fix the actual average cost of the care and keep of patients in the Hospital by considering the cost of ward patients, and by excluding any cost of patients using private rooms. The sum so arrived at shall be the cost of keeping a patient for this purpose, and no

part of the fund herein provided for shall be expended for the care and keep of any patient who actually pays a sum equal to the cost thus arrived at.

I realize that the sum given by me is not adequate to large work in all the lines herein suggested. My purpose in mentioning all of them is to give the Trustees of the Hospital the largest possible latitude in the expenditure of the income received from said fund that may be consistent with my desire that the same shall be used for the benefit of the deserving poor.

(6) Nothing in this deed of gift shall be construed as preventing a consolidation at any future time of the Medical Department of Northwestern University with one or more medical schools.

(7) The said fund is to be held, managed and controlled, with the power to sell, invest and reinvest, by the Board of Trustees of the Wesley Memorial Hospital. An annual audit of the books and accounts of the Hospital shall be made by a competent Public Accountant or Accountants, who shall also investigate and report on the condition of the fund, the income received therefrom and the expenditures made thereof, and especially shall they investigate and report as to whether or not such income has been applied in accordance with the conditions upon which this gift is made. A copy of such audit and report shall be published in the annual reports of the Hospital.

(8) If, at any time, any question of the interpretation of the terms of this deed of gift, or any question whatever arises under it and cannot be settled by the disagreeing parties, any three or more Trustees of Northwestern University, or any three or more Trustees of Wesley Memorial Hospital, may demand that the question at issue shall be referred in full detail to arbitration in the following manner: The committee above referred to of the University Trustees shall select one arbitrator; the committee above referred to of the Hospital Trustees shall select one arbitrator; the two arbitrators thus chosen shall select a third; and the majority decision of this arbitration committee shall be accepted by all parties in interest as final.

(9) This gift is to take effect upon the acceptance of the same and of the conditions specified by the Wesley Hospital, expressed by appropriate resolutions by its Board of Trustees, or by the Executive Committee thereof, and upon its changing its corporate name as specified; and also upon Northwestern University agreeing to all the conditions specified in this deed relating to its cooperation and affiliation with said Wesley Hospital, which agreement may be expressed by appropriate resolutions to that effect adopted by its Board of Trustees, or by the Executive Committee thereof.

IN WITNESS WHEREOF, I have hereunto set my hand and seal, this 9th day of April, A.D. 1914. Executed in duplicate copies.

(Signed) James Deering (SEAL)

It is interesting to note the order of conditions set forth by James Deering. In essence, he stipulated that:

(1) Wesley Hospital become a memorial to his father and sister.

(2) income from the fund be devoted to charity work; the Hospital should determine the needs of charity patients; Wesley should reach out and relieve unreported cases of misery; and conduct public health education programs.

(3) the mutual advantages of affiliation of Wesley Memorial Hospital and Northwestern University be maintained through a committee composed of an equal number from each institution including Northwestern University President, Dean of the medical department and an appointed Trustee; Wesley Hospital President, Superintendent and an appointed Trustee. The Northwestern representatives would serve on the Wesley board and the Wesley representatives would serve on the Northwestern board.

(4) the Hospital provide proper teaching facilities consistent with the principle that the patient's welfare be the first consideration; the Medical School provide adequate staff for the Hospital.

(5) income from the fund be used to care for the deserving poor only.

(6) the Medical School be free to consolidate with one or more medical schools.

(7) the fund be held, managed and controlled with power to sell, invest and reinvest by the Wesley Board of Trustees; the fund be audited annually and published in the Hospital's Annual Report.

(8) in the event of disagreement between the Hospital and Medical School each should choose an arbitrator and they should choose a third; the majority decision of the three-member committee would be final.

(9) the gift take effect upon acceptance of conditions specified and appropriate resolutions be adopted by both institutions.

Deering stressed the care and welfare of charity patients, the mutual advantages of hospital/university affiliation and even devised a means of arbitration should differences occur. He did not, however, consider the autonomous attitude of some physicians, educators and policy-making trustees. Authoritative traits in representatives of both participating institutions would misinterpret the donor's intent in years to come.

Forebodings   Chapter 10

If James Deering's satisfaction in his 1914 gift to Wesley was marred by the beneficiaries' discord, his enthusiasm for his second project, creating his new home, Vizcaya, was said to have prolonged his life. In 1910 James Deering, 51 years old and suffering from pernicious anemia, had homes in Chicago, Evanston, New York and Paris. While in residence in New York, he had met Paul Chalfin, an artist who had visited the great villas of Italy, whom Deering invited to accompany him to Europe to purchase furnishings and objets d'art for a new home. Mr. Deering collected statues, fountains, grilles, mantles, furniture, tapestries and carpets to be shipped to a New York warehouse.

Deering's Southern Home

Sharing his father's fondness for south Florida, James Deering purchased 130 acres of hummock and black marsh land on the shore of Biscayne Bay December 31, 1912. Until his home was erected, Deering rented a house in the area from Arthur Curtis James; his nearest neighbor was William Jennings Bryan.

Deering engaged E. Burrall Hoffman, Jr., an architect skilled in using old objects in new ways, to draw the plans. The estate had a private harbor with a massive stone barge decorated with sculpture by A. Stirling Calder, father of the sculptor, Alexander Calder. A gondola canal wound its way through the grounds which contained a lake, two tea houses, 25 miles of roadways and paths, as well as ten acres of Italian Renaissance gardens. The splendid four-tower, 70-room house of stucco and stone with red tile roofs was Italian in style with interior decor subtly combined with French.

Vizcaya, like Wesley, Opened Christmas Day

Mr. Deering's dream mansion was completed in December, 1916. On Christmas Day, a few friends and members of the family gathered for a housewarming at Vizcaya. It was a coincidence that this important day for James Deering was the 28th anniversary of the founding of Wesley Hospital, which had received its first patient on Christmas Day, 1888. One of Deering's early house guests at Vizcaya was the Reverend J. Shelley Meyer who, 28 years earlier, had carried Wesley's first patient from a taxicab to a bed in the Chicago Training School for Foreign Missions, founded and run by Meyer and his wife. He had served for years on Wesley's board, had been its superintendent twice and currently was vice president. He was able to report firsthand the growing tension between the Hospital and the University to their mutual benefactor.

Initiating Changes

Immediately after receiving the gift, Wesley began making alterations and adding services needed to comply with the Deering stipulations. A marble medallion, 29 inches in diameter, with the classic profiles of William Deering and his daughter, Abby Deering Howe, carved in bas-relief, was unveiled in the hospital lobby.

Charity work was increased from 28 percent in 1913 to 42 percent (31 percent free and 11 percent part pay) in 1915, or 2,632 of the 5,822 patients admitted during the year. In round numbers, free care expense was $60,400, of which $35,600 was income from the Deering fund. The churches contributed $10,000 and the Hospital gave $12,400 from its regular endowment and $2,400 from its earnings. The additional work intensified the need for social service to check the merits of indigent patients as directed in the Deering deed of gift, and to assist with family problems and follow-up care. The department was established in 1915 and within two years was handling about 7,000 social service visits and conferences annually.

Mrs. Sarah Wheeler, or "Aunt Sarah" (see page 49), donated her home and surrounding grove (valued at $20,000) in Lake Bluff for patients who were able to leave the Hospital, but still in need of nursing care. It was named the Wheeler Convalescent Home in memory of the donor's husband, the late George Wheeler.

The Ladies Aid Society had changed its name in 1915 to the Ladies Aid Auxiliary of Wesley Memorial Hospital (four years later it became the Woman's Auxiliary Board). The membership had grown to about 400 devoted women who served in many areas of the Hospital. Since the new building opened they had provided five drinking fountains, and garments to cloth indigent children when discharged, and had continued the annual tag day which raised about $2,500 annually for the children's ward. Their April, 1916 meeting was held in the Hospital's long-awaited new chapel, for which the women had provided the Bible and hymnals. Although they met in the Hospital, churches and various homes, their favorite rendezvous was the home of their president, Mrs. George W. Dixon, at 2706 South Michigan Avenue, the then fashionable boulevard lined with stone and brick mansions with tree-shaded gardens.

DIFFERENT POINTS OF VIEW

Wesley's expanded service, made possible by the Deering gift, was implemented despite the burden of its ongoing dispute with Northwestern University. In retrospect, the conflict between the Hospital and Medical School was inevitable. Their origin, organization, officers, personnel and purposes were different. It oversimplifies the issue to state that the Hospital was primarily interested in the care of its patients and the Medical School in the education of its students. More knowledge, experience and understanding would be required before the two factions could be reconciled.

WESLEY'S GOVERNING BOARD

The Hospital had been founded by medical, clerical and civic leaders to meet a grave community need, i.e. provision of hospital care for the sick poor. To this purpose, the members of the Board of Trustees who were legally responsible for the Hospital's operation had donated their time, experience and money. They were successful, conservative men of integrity with profound respect for the ideologies of their fathers. Their trusteeship was more than a moral and legal responsibility; it was a sacred trust.

Wesley president, Perley Lowe, had joined the board in 1894, only five years after the Hospital was founded, and had donated his services to several administrative functions including that of auditor. After discovering serious bookkeeping discrepancies which had adversely affected Wesley, he was persuaded in 1904 to accept the presidency and had been reelected each succeeding year.

The vice president in 1913, the year preceding the Deering gift, was Oliver H. Horton, prominent Chicago lawyer and judge of the Circuit Court, who had served as a Methodist delegate to an Ecumenical Conference in London in 1881. Eugene S. Gilmore had resigned as superintendent of the University of Michigan Hospital at Ann Arbor in 1908 to fill the same position at Wesley and to become a member of its Board of Trustees. The bylaws stipulated that ten of the 30 trustees be members of the Methodist Church.

Nine trustees formed the Executive Committee, which met quarterly and at special meetings called by the president. The committee was empowered by the bylaws to make contracts with agents and employees, to appoint the medical staff and fill vacancies, to elect a superintendent and to appoint interns from nominations of the medical staff. All matters of importance were reported and recommendations made and voted on at the annual meeting of the Board of Trustees, which was held on the third Saturday in January.

NORTHWESTERN'S MEDICAL COUNCIL

Northwestern University Medical School had a Medical Council consisting of the president (chief executive officer) and vice president of the University, dean of the Medical School, secretary of the medical faculty and others appointed annually by the Board of Trustees of the University. The medical faculty members were mostly practicing physicians who also taught classes and attended to administrative functions. Matters affecting the entire University were brought before the Executive Committee of its Board of Trustees.

In contrast to the continuous service of Wesley's board members, Northwestern's leaders changed frequently. Within the twenty years between 1905 and 1925 Northwestern University had three deans and two acting deans of the Medical School; five presidents of the Board of Trustees and four presidents of the University. The deans were Dr. Nathan S. Davis, Jr., 1901-1907; Dr. Arthur R. Edwards, 1907-1916; Dr. Arthur I. Kendall[1] (acting dean, 1916), 1917-1924; and Dr. James P. Simonds (acting dean 1924-1925). Dr. Davis and Dr. Kendall, the school's first full time dean, served on the Wesley board during their time in office. The presidents of the Board of Trustees were William Deering, 1897-1906; William F. McDowell, 1906-1917; James A Patten, 1917-1920; Oliver T. Wilson, 1920-1924, and Robert W. Campbell, 1924-1930. Presidents of the University were Thomas Franklin Holgate, 1904-1906, 1916-1919; Abram Winegardner Harris, 1906-1916; Lynn Harold Hough, 1919-1920, and Walter Dill Scott, 1920-1939.

The deans were comparatively young men who were either founders or alumni (except Dr. Kendall) of the school. Until 1916 private patients were their source of income. Dr. Edwards was 40 years old when he replaced Dr. Davis who was 49. Dr. Kendall was 39 when he became acting dean.

The deans' counterpart at Wesley was Eugene S. Gilmore, superintendent, who was appointed chief executive officer in 1908 and remained until his death in 1931 at the age of 61. Wesley president, Perley Lowe, had participated in the Hospital's day-to-day activities since becoming a trustee in 1894 at the age of 49. He had been a personal friend of William Deering and of his son, James. The two Wesley officers, Lowe and Gilmore, served through the tenures of Northwestern's 14 presidents of the Board of Trustees, the University, deans and acting deans in the controversial years.

Carnegie-AMA Report by Flexner

A report that would influence medical schools nationally and thereby affect hospitals had been made in 1907 when the American Medical Association's Committee on Improvement of Medical Education divided 240 medical schools into three classes: A, acceptable; B, doubtful; and C, unacceptable. The Northwestern Medical School was among 82 schools in Class A. Forty-six were B and 36 were C. Following the classifications, Abraham Flexner, a Johns Hopkins graduate who did advanced studies at Harvard and the University of Berlin, made inspections which were published in 1910 by the Carnegie Foundation jointly with the AMA. Among the

---

[1] *Dr. Kendall was not a physician; he was a graduate of Massachusetts Institute of Technology with doctorates in bacteriology from Johns Hopkins and in public health from Harvard University.*

weaknesses of medical education reported were lax admission requirements, poor financial support and lack of beds controlled by the medical schools. The report favored conditions at the richly endowed Johns Hopkins University, where admission required a baccalaureate degree and students were taught by a salaried faculty whose members also served as chiefs of the university hospital's departments and staff. About 70 medical schools closed immediately after the classifications. In Illinois, of 39 medical schools operating in 1909, only five remained open by 1926. The long-term result of the study was the reduction of 161 medical colleges throughout the country to 79.

Entrance requirements at Northwestern had been established in 1908 at one year of college preparation and were advanced to two years of college in 1911. The resulting decrease in enrollment was even more severe than had been predicted. From 599 medical students in 1908, the number dropped to 187 by 1914. This created a precarious condition in a school that depended on student fees as its main financial resource.

The Carnegie report emphasized that "a hospital under complete educational control is as necessary to a medical school as is a laboratory of chemistry or pathology." In the section on Northwestern, the patients available for students' clinical experience were considered varied and adequate. With Wesley's 80 free beds and additional ones at Mercy and Cook County hospitals, there were more beds available for teaching than could be used effectively. However, Northwestern was deficient in financial resources and it did not have complete control of the beds.

NORTHWESTERN'S ULTIMATUM

A letter addressed to the President and Board of Trustees of Wesley Memorial Hospital, signed by William F. McDowell, president of the Board of Trustees of Northwestern University and dated September 22, 1914, was received by the Hospital six months after its million dollar memorial gift from James Deering. The letter follows:

Gentlemen:

By direction of the Executive Committee of the Board of Trustees of Northwestern University, we beg to call your attention to the condition in the deed to the site of the Wesley Hospital building from Northwestern University dated June 30th, 1899, which deed is recorded in the office of the Recorder of Deeds of Cook County, Illinois, October 30th, 1899:

"This conveyance is made upon the express condition that said Wesley Hospital, the grantee herein, shall erect a Hospital building on said lot within a reasonable time, costing not less than $150,000, and maintain and operate said hospital, and that the staff of said hospital be drawn from faculties of Northwestern University Medical Schools and that facilities for clinic teaching be afforded the students of these schools in the wards and amphitheatre of the hospital as required by the grantor herein, and that on the failure of said Wesley Hospital to carry out these conditions, the title shall revert to Northwestern University."

Yesterday,...the Executive Committee learned that the Bylaws of Wesley Hospital which formerly read as follows:

"The Executive Committee is also empowered to make contracts with agents and employees, and to appoint annually the medical staff of the Hospital, on the nomination of such staff to be annually made by the Northwestern University, and they are empowered to fill vacancies in the same as they may arise, on similar nomination, by the Northwestern University," was changed and now reads as follows:

"The Executive Committee is also empowered to make contracts with agents and employees, and to appoint the Medical staff of the Hospital, and they are empowered to fill vacancies in the same as they may arise."

If it is intended by your Board that this change or amendment shall alter, modify or in anywise affect the condition in the deed mentioned and above quoted, we beg to inform you that such action on your part, or any course that may be taken by you in pursuance of such amended bylaw, or new paragraph as quoted above, is in violation of and contrary to the condition in the deed as quoted above, and such modification or amendment is not and cannot be assented to or acquiesced in by Northwestern University in anywise whatever.

In order that the said bylaw shall be perfectly clear...it is the judgment of the Trustees of the University that the original bylaw above quoted and long in force should be reinacted and the medical staff organized and if necessary reorganized in accordance with these conditions...

It is particularly requested that you strike from your medical staff the names of any and all physicians and surgeons not drawn from the faculties of the medical school or schools of Northwestern University, and discontinue service or services to any and all physicians and surgeons not so drawn, and give service only to such members of the faculties as may be designated by Northwestern University.

We beg also to say that in the opinion of the Executive Committee of Northwestern University, the action of the Board of Trustees of Wesley

Hospital in amending the Bylaw herein referred to, and any appointment or appointments made in pursuance of such amended bylaw heretofore or hereafter made, are in conflict with the spirit if not the letter of the deed of gift of Mr. James Deering to Wesley Hospital, dated April 9th, 1914, which in so far as it related to Northwestern University in imposing conditions upon it and upon Wesley Hospital was accepted by Northwestern University with the full understanding and expectation that Wesley Hospital, or Wesley Memorial Hospital, as the name now is, would willingly and cheerfully comply with the condition in the deed first hereinbefore mentioned and quoted.

Unless within twenty (20) days herefrom, your Board of Trustees or the Executive Committee thereof shall take steps to comply with the requests hereinabove stated, Northwestern University shall take such steps to protect its interests as the Executive Committee of its Board of Trustees shall deem fit and proper.

> Respectfully submitted,
> Northwestern University
> By (signed) William F. McDowell
> President of its Board of Trustees

APPROVED:
(signed) George T. Merritt
Attorney for the Board of Trustees
of Northwestern University

Mr. Deering Intervenes

The threat of litigation could be expected to invoke the diplomatic intervention of James Deering; and it did. Deering advised the boards of trustees of the dissenting institutions to invite Henry E. Pritchett, president of the Carnegie Foundation, to make a thoroughgoing study of both the Hospital and the Medical School and their relations. He accepted and, at the outset, displayed a clarity of vision that hostility had obscured in the conflicting parties.

Carnegie Report by Pritchett

A report addressed to the presidents of the governing boards of Wesley Memorial Hospital and Northwestern University, dated January 11, 1915, stated in part:

"It does not take a trained expert to appreciate that the two things which stand in the way of a prompt settlement of the existing differences are:

"1. A wide difference in the view of those who control the hospital and those who control the medical school as to what a hospital ought to be and how it ought to be conducted. Just so long as each of these views is insisted upon, no closer co-operation is likely. Two men who continue to look out of opposing windows are not going to see the same things no matter how honest each of them may be.

"2. The whole situation has become so complicated with personal feeling between the trustees and officers of the hospital and those of the medical school that a calm and fair consideration of the common problems is difficult. Unless the intensity of feeling can in some way be softened, no expert advice is going to improve the situation.

"The Wesley Memorial Hospital was by its charter intended 'For the gratuitous treatment of the medical and surgical diseases of the sick poor.' In the last annual report a somewhat different view of its purpose is given in the following language: 'Wesley Memorial Hospital is an institution of the Methodist Episcopal Church for the purpose of providing care for the sick, without regard to race or creed.' These two statements give a fair idea of the purpose of the hospital as it is framed in the minds of the trustees of that institution...Great attention is paid to securing patients and the greater part of the support comes from that source. The hospital is today indeed not so much a place for treatment of the sick poor as for the treatment of those who can pay, the profits from the latter, however, going for the use of the poor patients. Incidentally the hospital desires to offer facilities for medical teaching. Its obligations to do this are enormously increased by the acceptance of Mr. Deering's noble endowment. It does not afford at this time the opportunities for medical teaching which it ought to offer to the medical school.

"In comparison with this idea, the authorities of the medical school have in mind a hospital which shall care for the sick, whether rich or poor, but which shall use all of the material, so far as it will allow itself to be used, for teaching purposes. In order to carry out such a conception, it is necessary that the staff of the hospital shall be made up from the faculty of the medical school, and that when a teacher dissolves his connection with the medical school he should cease, ipso facto, to be a member of the hospital staff."

Mr. Pritchett explained that the arrangement was not yet possible at Northwestern's medical school which was not completely a university school of medicine, but was in a state of transition from a practitioner school where teachers served without pay. Northwestern clinical and surgical professors donated such time as they could afford from private practices. This created a situation in which medical practice was hopelessly confused with the claims of the medical school and of the hospital.

"The time will unquestionably come when the chief work of the clinical teachers will be that of the medical school and the hospital, and their practice will be confined entirely to the hospital. The medical school should look towards that aim now," Pritchett advised. He claimed that the question was not whether the ideal hospital could be brought into right relations with a fully developed university medical school, but whether a hospital long established and operated as a charity institution could be transformed into the hospital of a university in which the faculty was in the transition stage. He was convinced that this transformation could not be effected in a month or a year, but that if the hospital and the medical school began at once to cooperate sympathetically, they could in three or more years be convinced to accept the ideal arrangements towards which Mr. Deering's gift was directed.

Added Responsibilities   Chapter 11

Wesley trustees and the administrative staff continued to expand services to meet requirements of the Deering Deed of Gift as well as to meet their obligations to the patients, physicians, employees, volunteers, churches and thousands of other contributors.

The increased patient census required a larger operational staff: more nurses, medical technicians, employees in dietary, housekeeping, laundry and other departments providing patient services. To meet the higher payroll, patient beds had to be filled or Wesley could not remain solvent despite income for charity patients from the Deering gift. Patients could be admitted only through the medical staff. Therefore, when vacancies occurred on the medical staff and the university failed to fill them, the beds for those physicians' patients remained empty. Wesley then permitted non-staff physicians to use the facilities, though they were not invited to join the staff.

The attitude and the stand taken by Wesley's governing board is revealed in correspondence between its chief exponents, James Deering, benefactor, and Perley Lowe, president, from which the following excerpts are quoted.

Lowe to Deering
Chicago, July 25, 1916

...I would suggest that you now call the attention of the University people to their part of the agreement wherein they promised to put in "a full time salaried dean." I believe if they will do this, I can bring about a settlement of our difficulties...The Hospital is doing the best work in its history. We have received a number of bequests and know of more that are coming from other sources...

Lowe to Deering
Chicago, Jan. 2, 1917

...The University has withdrawn many of its objections and demands which we considered impossible to comply with, and the new dean (Dr. Kendall) has taken hold of his job in good shape and feels sure that he and Mr. Gilmore can work together...The doctors tell me it is absolutely necessary for me to go away because of my bronchial trouble; I am leaving for Pasadena for two or three months. Please send any communication you wish to make with the hospital to Mr. J. Shelley Meyer[1], vice president. While I am away, the whole matter will be in the hands of Vice President Meyer and the Executive Committee.

Lowe to Deering
Chicago, Jan. 10, 1917

...Saturday I was called on the telephone at midnight by the Chicago Tribune. They had prepared a long article in which there were a great many misstatements in regard to the Hospital and your request for the return of your million dollars. I should have been glad to have the whole matter suppressed but was unable to do so...I do not think that any of the trustees or anyone connected with the Hospital had anything to do with the matter...

The Sunday, January 7, 1917 issue of the *Chicago Tribune* carried the article referred to above in column 2 of the front page. The article shared equal space and headline type size with a front page story from the war front, "BRITISH DESTROY ENEMY TRENCHES UPON WIDE FRONT—Fierce Battles Are in Progress in France, Romania and Russia." The Wesley-Northwestern story was headed "DEERING WANTS BACK $1,000,000 HOSPITAL GIFT?—Dissatisfaction Over Wesley May Revive Northwestern U. Dispute." The text follows:

[1]*During this period, J. Shelley Meyer visited Mr. Deering at Vizcaya (page 70).*

The $1,000,000 from James Deering given early in 1914 to Wesley Memorial Hospital, Twenty-fifth and Dearborn streets, has revived the controversy of two years ago between the hospital and Northwestern university. It is reported that Mr. Deering is not satisfied with the administration of the hospital and through William J. Louderback, his business representative, he has intimated he would not refuse the return of his donation.

The gift of the million, which was in the nature of a memorial to Mr. Deering's father, William Deering, brought a hot debate between the trustees of Wesley hospital and the trustees of the university, the medical school of which is conducted in connection with the hospital.

Condition Made by Deering

Mr. Deering's gift named as one condition that the hospital should become a teaching hospital. The university authorities insisted this could be brought about only by permitting the medical school to appoint the staff of physicians, and to employ only physicians who were on the staff of the school.

At that time the matter seemed to be adjusted when Abram W. Harris, then president of Northwestern university said:

"The Wesley Memorial Hospital will be a teaching institution, and it is agreed the physicians and surgeons shall be chosen from the medical staff of the university, and a superintendent will be selected with authority over them."

Some Admit Deering Hint

"It is true that Mr. Louderback, business representative of Mr. Deering, spoke to me some few weeks ago in regard to Mr. Deering's million dollar donation," said Perley Lowe, president of the board of trustees of the hospital last night, "and that there was some intimation by Mr. Louderback that Mr. Deering would be willing to take back his gift.

"While no actual reasons were given for the intimation, it seems Mr. Deering is evidently not satisfied with the way things are being carried on. After my talk with Mr. Louderback I communicated with him, asking him to send the board of trustees a bill of particulars stating exactly what Mr. Deering's objections were. So far I have not heard anything more from him."

No Denial by Louderback

"If Mr. Lowe says that he had a conversation with me," said Mr. Louderback, "and that there was an intimation that Mr. Deering would be ready to accept the return of the million dollars which he donated, then Mr. Lowe must be right. That is all I have to say."

James Deering is in Florida and could not be reached last night.

Lowe to Deering

Chicago, March 26, 1917

Yours of the 17th followed me back from California. I note that you have consulted your attorney in this matter. I think if you ask for the return of your money on the grounds that you are not satisfied, there would be no opposition; but on the grounds that we have done anything wrong and have not lived up to the agreement in every respect, there would be a great deal of opposition. The trustees feel that the hospital has done exactly as it agreed...I do not know your present attorney but would like to meet him...I think there are a good many points on which you and he are not fully informed...The Hospital is prepared to give the school every assistance in its power and to receive every one of its doctors, but not allow them to manage or control the Hospital and consider it as part of their property or under their management...remember that the Hospital is a legally incorporated society which has thirty trustees who feel their responsibility of the trusts imposed upon them by their charter and by the many who have given to the Hospital...Therefore it is desirable, if possible, to find some solution; if not, for my own part, I shall favor returning your money...

Deering to Lowe

Vizcaya, Miami, March 31, 1917

...The attorney of whom I wrote you is one who was in the employ for many years of the Deering Harvester Company before consolidation. He is now again in the employ of the company which today, as you know, is the family firm for the investment and holding of property.

The best thing to be done surely is that you should make an appointment with Mr. Louderback and that Mr. McMath, the attorney, should be present. I can see very clearly the wisdom of your advice as to the form in which my request for the return of the money should be put and accordingly see the wisdom of consulting you before allowing any other kind of action to be taken...

Lowe to Deering

Chicago, April 4, 1917

...Now, as to meeting your Mr. McMath and Mr. Louderback, I will endeavor to do so very shortly...In the meantime, as you know, our country is on the verge of war, and all the resources at the command of the government are being canvassed...We had planned to turn over our Hospital to the government, so far as our facilities would permit...We have a building that was formerly a summer hotel at Lake Bluff, which has been donated to the Hospital. We could equip this to take care of fifty soldiers and could furnish the nurses and doctors. One of our nurses has recently returned from two years of service in the Allies Hospital in France and would be available to take charge...The hospital is now crowded to its full capacity...I have a letter from Mr. Meyer (J. Shelley Meyer, Wesley Vice President) which abounds with praise of your wonderful home and of the kind treatment you accorded him. He is quite familiar with matters here having run the Hospital himself...

Lowe to Deering
Chicago, Sept. 28, 1917
...In regard to the return of your money, I have personally advocated it at every meeting of the Executive Committee. I think to have it fully decided upon, it would have to go before the full Board of Trustees of the Hospital and of the University, as the University has notified us that they were interested in the matter and that they should be consulted before anything was done...

Lowe to Deering
Chicago, Jan. 18, 1918
...I had planned to bring a recommendation to the full Board of Trustees last Saturday that your money be returned to you...Mr. Merrick and one of Mr. Miller's partners, who, I understand are your attorneys, showed me the papers they proposed serving, of which I presume you are familiar...Both of these gentlemen told me that we could not legally return your money; it now belongs to the public. Other attorneys have since told me the same. Therefore I changed my plan and at the Board of Trustees meeting I verbally reported the facts and have referred the matter to the Executive Committee with power to act. They placed the matter in the hands of our attorney. I very much regret the way this matter has turned out. I have done my best to bring about an amicable settlement...

The letters reveal the paternal pride of Wesley trustees in their Hospital, their protective stand, hope for a reconciliation, then disappointment. The excerpts also depict James Deering's tact in his efforts to restore harmony and the trustees' resistance to demands they considered unjust.

Hostilities Abroad And at Home

Chapter 12

World War I had become a certainty on February 3, 1917, when the United States broke relations with Germany. Wesley doctors and nurses quickly responded when, on April 6, the United States declared war. Thirty of the Hospital's 63 attending and adjunct physicians and 13 of its 17 interns and fellows entered the armed forces.

In addition to caring for patients at home, the 37 remaining physicians served on the Medical Advisory Board of the Provost Marshal-General examining over 12,000 men to determine physical fitness for service. The hospital roof garden was used for this purpose. Those rejected were given medical and surgical attention, enabling many to join the armed forces later. Wesley gave free care to families dependent on service men.

One hundred Wesley alumnae, of whom 40 served overseas, answered the appeal of the American Red Cross for graduate nurses. One was sent to Romania, 14 to France, and 25 elsewhere in Europe; 50 worked in cantonments in the United States. Among those from Wesley's training school to enter the service were the head instructor of nurses and two administrative assistants. Others in key positions were the social service director, chief surgical nurse and head nurses on patient floors.

At the request of the Red Cross, Wesley women made 1,800 hospital gowns and pajamas for overseas use. Auxilians taught knitting to patients who, with physicians' approval, wished to participate. In one week ten pounds of yarn were knitted by patients and nurses, an achievement said to be the beginning of occupational therapy at Wesley.

The world-wide influenza epidemic of 1918 reached devastating proportions within Wesley. The very contagious viral disease, which killed an estimated five to ten million persons throughout the world in 1918 and 1919, struck 70 nurses at the Hospital. There were no fatalities, although several had not yet recovered when the war ended November 11, 1918.

WORLD WAR I ROLL OF HONOR
Wesley Medical Staff members of Base Hospital Unit Number 12, U.S. Army Medical Corps, which served in France, are listed under their hospital departments with army ranks when they entered the service. All are on the World War I Honor Roll of faculty and alumni of Northwestern University Medical School.

Medicine
Robert B. Preble, Lt. Col.
Arthur F. Byfield, Capt.
James Gray Carr, Capt.
Martin R. Chase, Maj.
William F. Holmes, Maj.
Walter H. Nadler, Maj.
Charles P. Horner, Capt.
Don C. Sutton, Capt.
Hugo W. Traub, 1st Lt.

Surgery
Allen B. Kanaval, Col.
Frederick A. Besley, Lt. Col.
Jacob R. Buchbinder, 1st Lt.
William R. Cubbins, Maj.
Sumner L. Koch, Maj.
William E. Shackleton, Capt.
Leslie H. Hills, 1st Lt.
John W. Miller, 1st Lt.

Gynecology
Payson L. Nusbaum, Maj.
Eugene Cary, 1st Lt.
Wesley J. Woolston, 1st Lt.

Obstetrics
David S. Hillis, Lt. Cmdr.
(U.S. Navy)
Charles B. Reed, 1st Lt.

Dermatology
Joseph S. Eisenstaedt, Lt.

Neurology
Lewis J. Pollock, Capt.

Nose and Throat
Frederick Menge, Maj.
Otis T. McClay, Capt.
Charles P. Younger, Capt.

Ophthalmology
George T. Jordan, Capt.

Oral Surgery
Herbert A. Potts, Maj.

Genito Urinary
Hugo E. Schmidt, 1st Lt.

Interns
James A. Washburn, Capt.
William E. Anspach, 1st Lt.
Harvey A. Feltz, 1st Lt.
Arthur J. Fletcher, 1st Lt.
Roy C. Hawthorne, 1st Lt.

Andrew J. Hedgecock, (Naval Reserve)
John W. Iddings, 1st Lt.
Francis Kleinman, 1st Lt.
Herman O. McPheeters, 1st Lt.
Fred Martin, 1st Lt.
Hiram Y. Richards, 1st Lt.
George J. Rivard, 1st Lt.
Cyril Amos Youngs (Naval Reserve)

Fellows
George Carl Fenn, Capt.
Charles P. Horner, Capt.
Willis S. Gibson, 1st Lt.

Northwestern Versus Wesley and Deering
More than half of Wesley's doctors were engaged in warfare abroad on February 6, 1918, when Northwestern University, complaintant, filed a bill in chancery against Wesley Memorial Hospital and James Deering, to enforce a charitable trust. M. W. Pinckney was the presiding judge. The bill was based upon the deed from Northwestern University to Wesley Hospital printed below in full, barring the legal description of the property, and certificates at the conclusion:

(U.S. Revenue Stamps to the amount of $20.00.)
This Indenture Witnesseth, That the Grantor, Northwestern University, a corporation existing under the laws of the State of Illnois, of the City of Evanston, in the County of Cook and State of Illinois, for and in consideration of the sum of One Dollar and other valuable consideration in hand paid, Conveys and Warrants to Wesley Hospital, a corporation existing under the laws of the State of Illinois, of the City of Chicago, County of Cook and State of Illinois, the following described Real Estate to wit: (Legal description of property. Revenue stamps at the top indicate that the two lots were valued at $20,000.)
This conveyance is made upon the express condition that said Wesley hospital, the Grantee herein, shall erect a hospital building on said lot within a reasonable time, costing not less than $150,000, and maintain and operate said hospital, and that the staff of the hospital be drawn from the

faculties of Northwestern University Medical School and that facilities for clinic teaching be afforded the students of those schools in the wards and amphitheater of the hospital, as required by the grantor herein, and that on the failure of said Wesley Hospital to carry out these conditions the title shall revert to Northwestern University.

Dated, this thirtieth day of June, A.D. 1899.

Northwestern University, (Seal.)
By William Deering, President.

Northwestern claimed that eminent physicians on the university faculty, properly recommended, were not admitted to Wesley's staff; that unqualified members dropped from the medical faculty had been retained on the hospital staff over the school's protests. It accused Wesley of changing its bylaws to omit a university privilege, the right to nominate staff appointments, after the original signing of the property deed. The University alleged that Wesley provided less than six percent of clinical experience required for the students and that they were not admitted to patient wards. The Wesley superintendent was criticized as being disinterested in the scientific part of medical education and his dismissal was recommended.

WESLEY'S POINT OF VIEW

The Carnegie Foundation president, Henry S. Pritchett, had said in appraising the situation, "Two men who continue to look out of opposing windows are not going to see the same things no matter how honest each of them may be." Wesley trustees continued to view the conflict from their window and Northwestern trustees continued to judge the discord from their side.

Wesley president, Perley Lowe, summarized the Hospital's grievances in its 30th Annual Report, printed and distributed in 1919 to its public— persons associated with Wesley and its thousands of donors and friends. The President's Report is printed in part below:

Chicago, January 18, 1919

". . . You will remember that in the deed of our property from Northwestern University occurs the following clause: (see deed of conveyance, page 86).

"We agreed to draw our staff from the faculty of Northwestern University, and we have never drawn anyone who was not a member of that faculty. In return the University was to furnish us an adequate staff; this they have never done...therefore, we have had to depend on outside doctors for patients to fill our rooms and wards.

"For many years the University took very little interest in the Hospital. After we had cleared the Hospital of debt, and built and paid for a new wing, it became more attractive to the University and there was evinced a desire to control the Hospital...Friction grew out of this situation, and the University threatened us with legal proceedings based on the clause above mentioned. Doctors who had long been on the University faculty and members of our staff were summarily dismissed from the University faculty and we were then directed to dismiss them from our staff. They were among our most faithful and useful members and we owed them gratitude for helping us through the dark days of financial depression and so declined to acquiesce...Numerous conferences were held to bring about a friendly agreement, but none of these assured willingness to compromise.

"The day of our annual meeting a year ago an attorney for the University served notice of their intention to appeal to the courts. I laid the paper before the trustees and was directed to defend their suit...

"The suit was heard in the Circuit Court...Judge Pinckney dismissed the case for lack of jurisdiction and equity. They (Northwestern) quite likely will appeal to the Supreme Court...Inasmuch as the University has gone to the courts to have this matter settled, we are desirous that it be settled for all time.

It is our intention and desire, whatever the result, to carry out the original intentions and wishes of Mr. Deering; to be helpful to the medical school in every way, having in mind that we must maintain the interests of the patient and the Hospital."

Respectfully,
Perley Lowe, *President*

CARE AND TEACHING CONTINUE

The law suit did not prevent the complainant (Northwestern University) or the defendant (Wesley Memorial Hospital) from continuing their interdependent programs of treating sick patients and teaching medical students.

The Wesley Annual Report distributed in 1921 revealed that the Deering Fund provided $53,784.48 of the $76,461.80 spent for free care during the preceding year. "The funds were administered in strict accordance with the agreement made with Mr. Deering," Perley Lowe stated in his presidential report. Of Wesley's 1,291 charity patients, the costs of 831 were met by the Deering Fund in 1920. The medical care was given

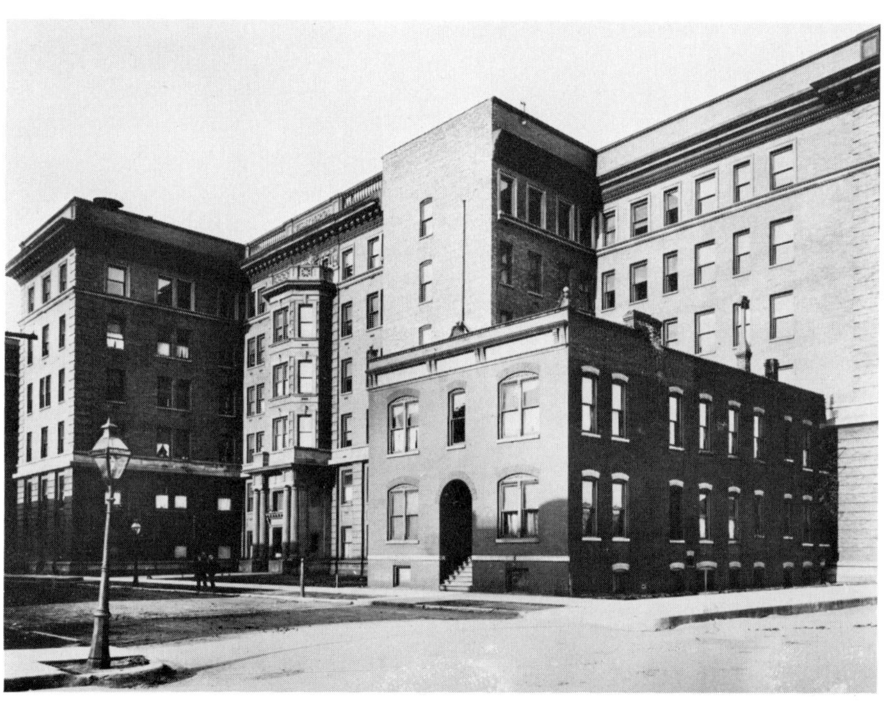

Wesley's six-story steel and brick building for 181 patients opened in June, 1901. The small structure in foreground was used until 1910, then razed.

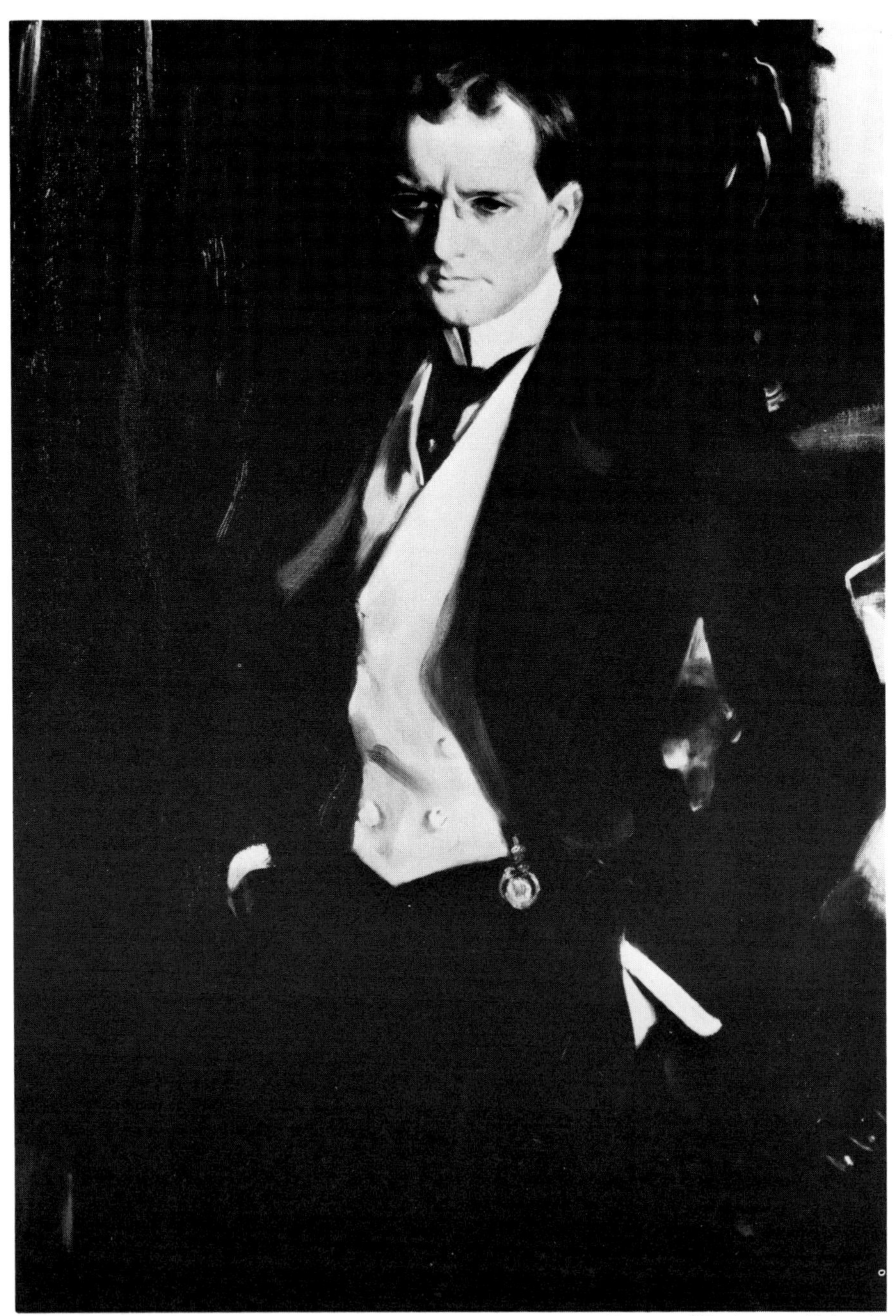

*James Deering, 1858-1925, memorialized
his father and sister through a million
dollar gift to Wesley for teaching and
charity purposes.*

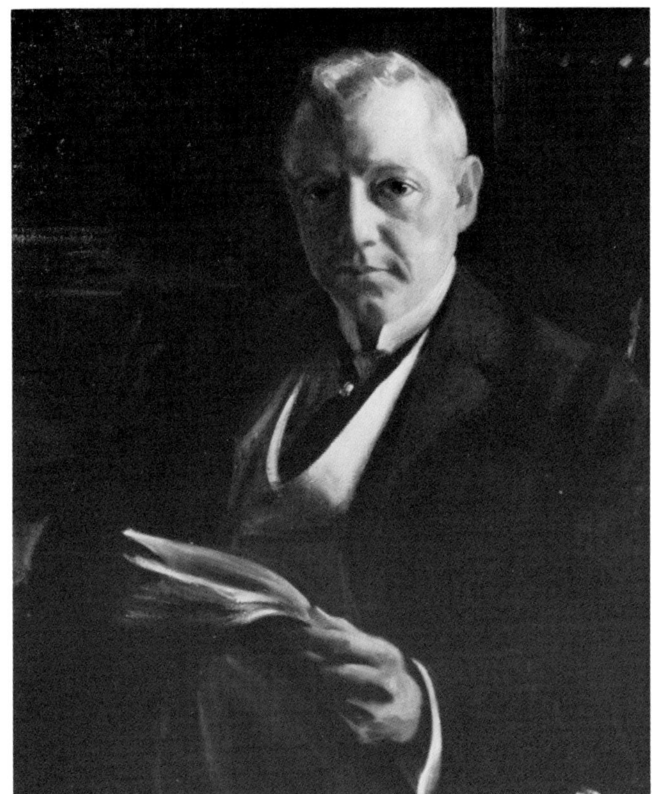

Courtesy of Northwestern University

Charles Deering continued the family philanthropic pattern until his death in 1927. Deering donations equaled a grand total of $1,870,000.

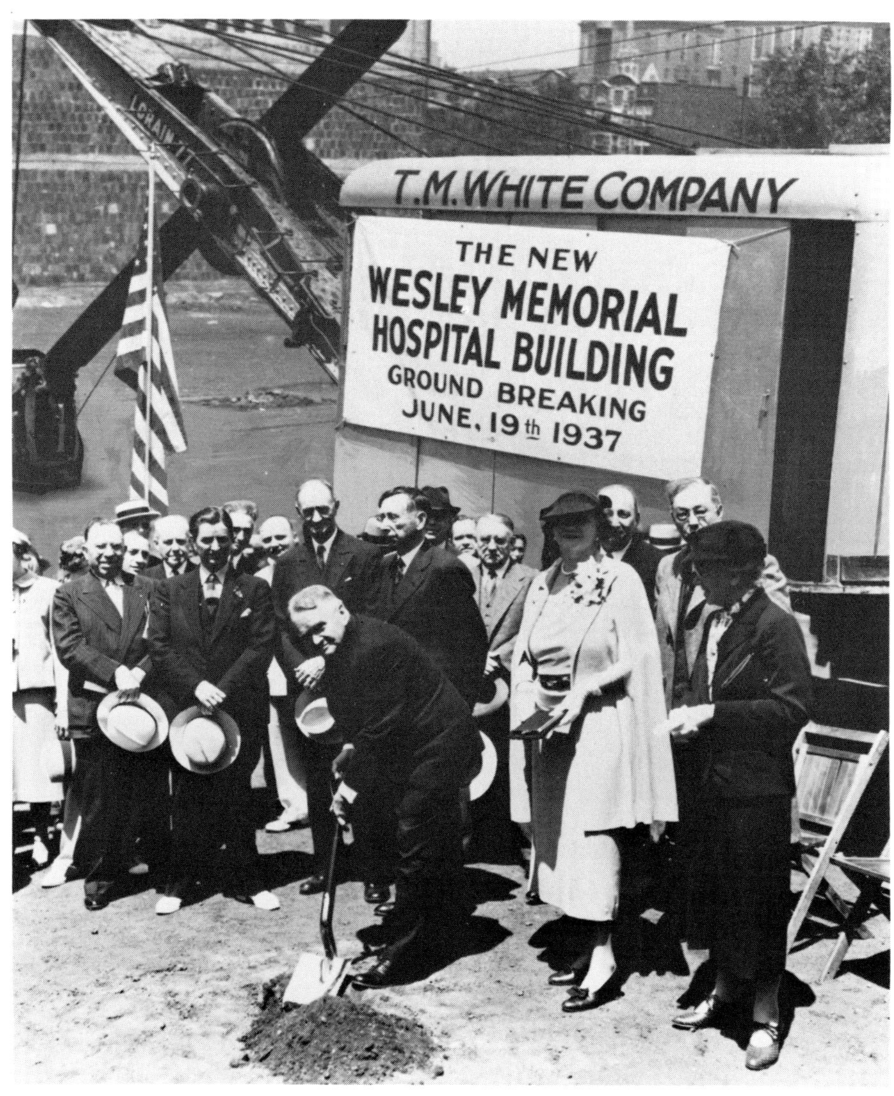

*George Herbert Jones, three million dollar
donor, turned the first spadeful of earth
for Wesley's new home on NU's near
north campus.*

gratuitously by the Wesley medical staff. The Hospital's chief of staff was Dr. William E. Schroeder; the staff secretary was Dr. Charles A. Elliott, chairman of Northwestern's department of medicine 1917-1939.

Wesley had increased its diagnostic services in 1920 by installing laboratories for physiological chemistry and electrocardiographic work. The x-ray department had been equipped both for diagnosis and deep therapy. The Hospital had accumulated $50,000, which was applied to a $100,000 land purchase of 450 feet of frontage on the west side of Dearborn Street across from the Hospital. Plans had been drawn for a nurses' residence on the new property.

A FRIENDLY SUIT

The controversy seemed to have reached an impasse in 1922 and no one could predict its end. James Deering paraphrased Mr. Pritchett's analogy when he wrote in a letter dated March 20, 1923 to Perley Lowe: "Two persons cannot always see the same question in the same light. I am sure I have never had the slightest doubt that your position in the question between the Hospital and the University has been conscientiously and carefully considered. I am sure that you will give me credit for the same spirit.

"As far as I am concerned the law suit that has occurred and is still going on might well be called a friendly suit. I have always respected you as my father's good friend, and in later years have felt that you were also my friend. As you know, I modified the language of the deed of gift out of this consideration..."

RECOGNITION OF HOSPITAL ADMINISTRATION

A factor not generally considered by medical schools in the quest for control of hospital beds was the development of hospital administration. In September, 1899, the year Wesley agreed to affiliate with Northwestern, eight men—four from Cleveland, two from Detroit and one each from Ann Arbor and Pittsburgh—met in Cleveland and formed the Association of Hospital Superintendents. This was the first move toward recognition of hospital administration as an independent profession separate from medical science. Previously, administration, for the most part, had been conducted by trial and error, sometimes without preparation or plan. Need for the new organization was confirmed by its swift growth to 234 member superintendents by 1906 when its name was changed to the American Hospital Association (AHA) of the United States and Canada.

The program of the annual AHA convention in 1907, the first one held in Chicago, listed among the interesting papers to be presented, "Organization of a Teaching Hospital," by Eugene S. Gilmore; "Employees and Their Selection and Management-Comparison of Hospital Payroll," by Asa S. Bacon; "Report of a Subcommittee on Hospital Services, Hospital Finance and Economics of Administration," by Dr. Sigismund S. Goldwater. All three authors distinguished themselves in service to hospitals and each became president of the AHA; Goldwater, 1908, Bacon, 1923, and Gilmore, 1925.

Eugene S. Gilmore, who had served as superintendent of the University of Michigan Hospital at Ann Arbor for nine years, had accepted the same position at Wesley as its first full time paid administrator, taking office April 1, 1908. He also served the community as a trustee of the Chicago Hospital Association, Northwestern University, and Wesley.

On the broader scale, Mr. Gilmore was the first president of the Methodist Hospital Association; secretary of the Board of Hospitals, Homes and Deaconess Work of the Methodist Episcopal Church; trustee of the Protestant Hospital Association and trustee, vice-president, and president of the American Hospital Association. His many honors reflected credit upon his hospital. When Northwestern insisted that Gilmore be terminated as superintendent of the Hospital and replaced by a dean of the medical school, the Wesley trustees declined.

THE OPINION OF THE JUDGE

Northwestern's suit did go to the Illinois Supreme Court along with a brief and argument prepared for Wesley Memorial Hospital and James Deering, submitted February 3, 1919, by Wesley's attorneys, N. M. Jones, Archibald Cattell and E. Allen Frost. The allegations in Northwestern's suit and the counterevidence in Wesley's rejoinder were reviewed and discussed. The opinion of Judge Pinckney, delivered October 3, 1918, was appended to the brief; excerpts are quoted below.

> "I cannot see anything in this case from the papers and the law as cited but
> that the bill is obnoxious to this general demurrer, absolutely...In my

opinion, the rights of the Northwestern University and the Wesley Memorial Hospital were absolutely fixed and determined back in 1899 when the Wesley Memorial Hospital...accepted the gift to the extent that they built the building and spent, with or without the thirty thousand dollars[1], one hundred and fifty thousand dollars. The moment that its rights became fixed there was nothing any court could do 14 years later, either by hooking it up with this deed of gift, to which they were entitled to have compliance in a proper case or by associating together these two deeds of gift, in order to hold this case in a court of chancery...

"I cannot see it in any other light. James Deering, when he made his deed of gift in 1914 fully cognizant of all these conditions and of this trouble, had he intended to do anything but that which he expressed in his deed of April 9, 1914, he would have said so, in my opinion. When he does not say so, being cognizant or familiar with those conditions and that trouble, he leaves a court to determine from the conditions of his gift, what to do and how it should be administered. It is not necessary for this court to tell any one of you gentlemen what you can do...The only order necessary to enter in this case is an order sustaining the demurrer to the bill, dismissing it for want of equity. That order you may prepare."

THE SETTLEMENT

The demurrer was sustained until the end of Wesley's 35th year when a settlement was reached that was satisfactory both to the Hospital and the University. Northwestern, having acquired land for a Chicago campus east of Michigan Avenue, was seeking funds for buildings; it requested an end to the quarrel in order to approach influential friends of both institutions.

In the Hospital's Annual Report for 1923-1924, Superintendent Gilmore announced in his section that "the long-standing difficulties between Northwestern University and Wesley Memorial Hospital have been settled amicably and with honor and advantage to both institutions." The provisions were: (a) erection of at least a 400-bed hospital by Wesley on the new campus; (b) not less than one-third[2] of the total bed capacity be allocated to patients available for progressive clinical instruction; (c) the Hospital to select its staff exclusively from the University faculty although current non-faculty members could remain (severance from the faculty not

[1]*The school had given the hospital $30,000 shortly after affiliation.*

[2]*In 1929 the bed allocation was reduced from 133 to 15 at all times, plus others supported by specific endowments.*

necessarily to mean severance from the hospital staff); (d) contemporaneously with execution of contract of affiliation, Northwestern to convey to Wesley all interest in its present property, to release all claims against the Hospital arising out of any gifts, dismiss the bill and cross-bill without cost to any party thereto; (e) Wesley to allot at least 50 beds for clinical instruction until erection of new hospital (both parties observe all conditions of the Deering gift); if Wesley desires to build on the new campus, Northwestern to provide a site of about 30,000 square feet adjoining the school at a nominal rental.

Thus the ten-year battle was legally ended, but the true spirit of friendship and cooperation which William Deering had insisted upon and which his son, James, had endeavored to bring about, was yet to come.

The Aftermath   Chapter 13

During the Wesley/Northwestern negotiations which had brought about the legal settlement, James Deering's health had begun to fail rapidly. The pernicious anemia had so weakened him that he used a wheelchair to go into his gardens for fresh air and, in early 1925, he required several blood transfusions. However, he rallied enough to make his annual visit to Paris before his condition became critical. He expressed an intense desire to return home and was carried, in a coma, aboard the S. S. Paris. He died September 21, 1925, without recovering consciousness, during a storm off the coast of Newfoundland.

James Deering's benevolence had extended to those less fortunate wherever he happened to be. He had willed $500,000 to establish a ward[1] for male patients in Jackson Memorial Hospital at Miami where Vizcaya was located; again, in memory of his father, William Deering. His brother, Charles Deering, added $100,000 so that the income from $600,000 was, and still is, available annually for the care of indigent Miami patients.

James Deering bequeathed Vizcaya to his nephews and nieces, two of

----

[1]*The Deering Ward at Jackson Memorial Hospital was closed after a Supreme Court ruling that indigent patients may not be segregated from those who pay. Following court determination, the fund expends monies for nursing care of indigent patients and for capital equipment at the hospital, according to J. Deering Danielson, trustee for the Deering Fund. May, 1980*

whom, Marion Deering McCormick (Mrs. Chauncey McCormick) and Barbara Deering Danielson (Mrs. Richard Ely Danielson), daughters of Charles, purchased the interests of other heirs. They arranged to convey the mansion, art, furnishings, and entire estate to Dade County as a public museum, a permanent memorial to their uncle, James Deering.

Appropriately, the man who honored his father by providing health care for thousands, himself was commemorated by enriching others through public availability of the art and culture he loved. On February 5, 1927, less than two years after the demise of James Deering, his brother Charles, the last of William Deering's immediate family, died.

Charles Deering already had given the State Street property, valued at $160,000, to Wesley and he bequeathed $340,000, leaving a total of half a million for Wesley. William Deering had started the philanthropic pattern with $60,000 toward the land and original building, followed by $225,000 for endowment, $65,000 for the southwest building and $20,000 unallocated, amounting to $370,000. This, together with his sons' donations, equaled a grand total of $1,870,000.

The Hospital expressed its gratitude on December 14, 1927, when Mrs. Chauncey McCormick presented an oil painting of her uncle James by the noted French artist, Anders Zorn, which was placed near the marble medallion of William Deering and daughter, Abby Deering Howe. Mrs. McCormick gave Wesley a photograph of her father, Charles Deering, with the promise of a portrait later. The artist, Zorn, a personal friend of Charles Deering, painted the portrait which was hung next to that of his brother.

Wesley trustees agreed that without the benevolence of the Deering family, whose deep concern for its fellow man prompted such kind and generous acts, it is doubtful that Wesley Memorial Hospital could have achieved its prominence in the hospital field.

Loss of Other Friends
Several of Wesley's strong supporters who had dedicated their major efforts to the Hospital's work had died during the early years of the turbulent twenties. Lucy Rider Meyer, one of Wesley's founders, had died in the Hospital March 16, 1922. Her husband, Josiah Shelley Meyer, died of a stroke July 1, 1926. At the time of his death he was vice president of Wesley. Together, the Meyers and those they trained were founders of forty

welfare institutions. They also were pioneers in educating women for health service and other social work.

Mrs. Gustavus F. (Annie M.) Swift died May 19, 1922, 19 years after the death of her husband, who had become a trustee in 1896. Shortly before she succumbed Mrs. Swift had given $50,000 for a nurses residence and she had left another $50,000 to Wesley in her will.

Mrs. George (Aunt Sarah) Wheeler, Woman's Auxiliary president 1903-1904, Wesley trustee and devoted volunteer who had given her Lake Bluff estate for a convalescent home, died at Wesley from pneumonia February 15, 1923.

Perley Lowe, Wesley trustee since 1894, had been elected president in 1904, remaining in office until his death, July 29, 1924, in his 79th year. He had been a lumberman from Levant, Maine, who had come to Chicago in 1867, had been elected director, vice president and president of the Lumbermen's Exchange, and was a prominent layman of the Methodist Episcopal Church.

Death came to Mrs. George W. (Marion Martin) Dixon on January 4, 1926. She had served as president of the Woman's Auxiliary for 18 years and was known for her good works throughout the city. Mr. Dixon gave $20,000 to the Wesley Endowment Fund in his wife's memory.

Dr. William E. Schroeder, Wesley's chief of staff for the past decade, also died in 1926. He had recently presented his private medical library, valued at $25,000, to the Hospital he had served for 30 years.

OPTIMISTIC OUTLOOK

George William Dixon, second son of Arthur Dixon and trustee since 1914, was vice president when Perley Lowe died in 1924. Dixon assumed the office and was elected president at the next annual meeting. Other officers were Frederick John Thielbar, well-known architect, vice president; Edwin Levitt Wagner, bank president, secretary; M. Haddon McLean, banker, treasurer; Nathaniel Magruder Jones, lawyer, counsel; and Eugene S. Gilmore, hospital superintendent. Also listed as an officer was J.L. Anderson, D.D., corresponding secretary and chaplain, who had succeeded Miles Wilbur Satterfield, D.D., after his death in 1921.

Mr. Dixon's report dated January 17, 1925, revealed that for the first time in Wesley's history, the annual income passed the half million dollar mark. The 1924 income was $500,106.23 and the operating expenses were $445,477.68, leaving a surplus of $44,628.55. Of this amount, $11,266.63 was given to the free care fund leaving an operating surplus of $33,361.92. A number of recent gifts had increased the endowment fund to $436,169.92 excluding the million dollar Deering gift which remained intact. Patients admitted totaled 8,513 of whom 2,144 received free care at a cost of more than $94,000.

Northwestern University had procured land on the near north side of Chicago and had plans drawn for medical and dental schools. Beginning in December, 1923, Mrs. Montgomery Ward had contributed three munificent gifts totaling more than eight million dollars for Northwestern's medical and dental schools in memory of her husband, a Chicago civic leader and mail-order merchant.

Relative to Northwestern's building program, Dixon's 1925 report announced Wesley's purchase of land at the northwest corner of Superior Street with a 216-foot frontage, and Fairbanks Court with 125-foot frontage, at a cost of $225,000 to be given by the Methodist Book Concern. Northwestern had proposed to lease to Wesley at a nominal sum the adjoining property of 34,000 square feet provided that Wesley could erect a hospital building on the site by January 1, 1929. This was according to the new contract of affiliation with the Medical School when the Hospital agreed to erect a thoroughly modern hospital plant on or near the McKinlock Campus.

New Campus Honors McKinlock

The McKinlock Campus had been so named in appreciation for a $250,000 pledge to Northwestern in 1921 by Mr. and Mrs. George A. McKinlock in memory of their son, Alexander McKinlock, Jr., who was killed in France during World War I. In 1930, huge iron gates were installed at the campus entrance at Superior Street and Lake Shore Drive, said to be the largest wrought iron ornamental pieces ever created in the United States. Mr. McKinlock died December 16, 1936 and his estate was unable to meet the capital pledge. The following year the campus was renamed the Chicago Campus of Northwestern University. However, the gates remained to commemorate Alexander McKinlock's heroic action.

The Cost Spiral

In the president's report for 1927, Dixon compared the current cost per patient day, $9.37, to that of 1891 when the cost per patient day per capita was $1.00. He blamed the jump of more than 900 percent in 36 years on increased cost of supplies, higher wage scale and medical advances requiring highly scientific equipment operated by skilled technicians[1].

Mr. Dixon further disclosed that routine tests in 1891 were limited to blood counts and urinalyses performed in the pathological laboratory. The physiological chemistry laboratory of 1927 provided results that immeasurably improved diagnoses and treatment. The blood and metabolic laboratory established in 1920 had, seven years later, become the most complete department of its kind in Chicago for patients with conditions such as diabetes, nephritis, goiter and heart disease. Research at Wesley had revealed a new test for gallbladder and the enlarged x-ray department gave additional assistance to physicians in their diagnoses. Deep therapy for cancer had begun, a service that would expand to save thousands of lives. These and other innovations at Wesley aided medical science in its ascent to today's undreamed of success in extending human life—and the corresponding ascent of costs.

Clouds Gather

Wesley's optimism was short-lived for, along with financial success, Dixon's 1927 report conceded that "no satisfactory arrangements have been consummated between Wesley Hospital and Northwestern University...We have endeavored to enter into a ground lease with the University which would carry out and embody the purpose and intent of the contract of affiliation." He explained that the property lease submitted by the University contained the forfeiture provisions found in an ordinary commercial lease between landlord and tenant where parties deal with each other at arms' length and with suspicion. He pointed out that the value of the land to be leased was but a fraction of the investment the Hospital would make, therefore Wesley could not agree to a commercial ground lease with easy forfeitures. The Hospital then submitted a suggested lease without easy forfeitures which was refused. This contention continued for

[1]*Hospital people may reflect that during the past 50 years or more, hospital costs have risen in similar proportion and for the same reasons as those given by Dixon in 1927.*

two years while the Ward Building, the first to rise on the new campus, was completed for classes in the 1926-27 school year.

PROSPERITY IS REVERSED

So successful had been Wesley's service in patient care, research and education in the early 1920s that the gradual deterioration of its neighborhood had scarcely been noticed. More and more residents and established businesses were moving northeast, leaving the 25th Street and Dearborn Avenue area vacant for vagrants. As the slums closed in, paying patients became reluctant to enter the hospital and nurses were afraid to walk outside in the dangerous environment.

The Stock Market crashed in October of 1929, followed by the closing of over 37,000 banks, corporations and businesses throughout the country. The nation slid into the Great Depression, and Wesley was one of its victims. More and more patients sought Wesley's help but were unable to pay. Many annual donors no longer had money to give. Several members of the medical and nursing staffs changed to other hospitals in better locations and with stronger financial backing. Wesley faced a bleak future.

The Grim Decade   Chapter 14

The year 1930 ushered in a troublesome decade bracketed in history by the world's greatest depression and its most devastating war. As the Depression deepened, 12 million persons across the nation were said to be unemployed and the effects were felt at every level, particularly institutions supported by charity. A local reflection of poverty-induced penny-pinching occurred on Tag Day. Wesley was one of 50 Chicago health and welfare institutions which, since 1910, had benefited each October when volunteers at allotted tagging stations sought donations from passersby. Wesley's children's ward had received about $4,000 annually on tag day. The bitter disappointment of the Woman's Auxiliary in the meager results of the 1930 tagging was recorded by the secretary: "Dimes instead of quarters were dropped in the boxes; nickels instead of dimes; more frequently pennies in place of all three. There were seven thousand pennies in the receipts. The deficiency was not sustained by Wesley taggers only; it was suffered by all participating organizations."

Wesley was bereaved at the loss of Eugene Stuart Gilmore, its superintendent for 23 years, who died of a heart attack at his desk in the Hospital September 12, 1931. Under his guidance, Wesley was said to be one of the ten leading hospitals in the United States. After serving as president of the American Hospital Association in 1925, Gilmore had been a delegate to the International Congress of Christian Work in South America, later touring the country to study the Methodist missionary hospital program. Gilmore took special pride in the fact that of the 66 hospitals in Chicago, Wesley provided the largest share of free care.

In his last annual report, Gilmore stated that Wesley had admitted 5,437 patients, of whom 1,417 received free care. Of these, expenses for 720, or about half, were provided by the Deering Fund; the remainder came from churches and the endowment fund. However, the influx of medically indigent patients became so great that in 1931 each person in the free bed ward was asked to pay as much as he could, even if it was only $5. Gilmore was succeeded as superintendent by Paul H. Fesler, who also served as president of the American Hospital Association for the year 1932.

Chaplain J. L. Anderson, D.D. who had given counsel and spiritual strength to discouraged volunteers and employees as well as to patients during those troubled times, died in April, 1932.

SIGNS OF THE TIMES

An indication of internal dissatisfaction at Wesley was a separate column in the medical staff roster of the 1930 Annual Report preceded by: "Because of long and distinguished service in Wesley Memorial Hospital, the following doctors, now engaged elsewhere, have been enrolled as Emeritus Attending Men." Listed were Drs. James G. Carr, Archibald Church, Charles A. Elliott, Hugh T. Patrick, Robert Preble, Brown Pusey, Harry M. Richter and Frederick R. Zeit. By 1934 Drs. Sanford R. Gifford, Allen B. Kanavel, Otto S. Pavlik, Samuel C. Plummer, James P. Simonds, Frederick C. Test and John Gordon Wilson had been added to the list.

Effects of the Depression on occupancy were revealed in fiscal data. In 1927, 6,818 patients were admitted, of whom 1,924 were free or part pay. In 1928, patients admitted had decreased to 6,177 and free or part pay patients had increased to 1,972. The gap between free and paying patients continued to diminish. In 1932, the total number of admitted patients dropped to 3,776 and free patients totaled 1,424, or well over one third of all patients.

With only half of the beds occupied in 1933 the Hospital was forced to close several patient floors. The children's free bed ward was closed in 1934 because of a $2,000 monthly deficit. However, no child was refused admittance. Sick children were placed in unoccupied rooms on adult floors and almost as many received care in 1934 as in the preceding year.

Too Many Eggs

Patients sent in by relief organizations often were undernourished and required special diets, an added burden to the already-deficient dietary budget. The Woman's Auxiliary examined the problem and presented a project that focused on Easter, 1935, and continued for 22 years. The idea was initiated by the group's president, Mrs. William F. Dangel, and the delicacy committee chairman, Mrs. J. R. Richardson, who wrote to each woman's society in the 371 churches of the Rock River Conference requesting eggs for patients at Easter. In reply, 951 dozen eggs valued at $264.72 were received and the enterprise became an annual Lenten project.

Some churches supplemented eggs with cash, but the donors seemed to favor eggs. In 1945, 2,778 dozen or 33,336 individual eggs rolled into Wesley's kitchen. In its next request the Hospital implied that cash would be preferable. By 1957, when the Lenten season letter was discontinued, Wesley had received innumerable eggs and $27,733 in cash from its version of an annual Easter egg hunt.

School of Nursing is Closed

The Wesley School of Nursing became a Depression casualty when its doors were closed in 1935. The school's first graduates had been three deaconesses of the class of 1890 followed by approximately 1,000 nurses during the next 45 years. Under the direction of Bertha L. Knapp, principal of the school and superintendent of nursing at the Hospital since 1908, the school had developed an excellent training program which provided most of Wesley's nurses, and many for other areas requiring nurses. Seventeen alumnae served in foreign fields, 28 in public health, 60 in other hospitals, 10 as assistants in doctors' offices, 12 in industrial plants and 224 in private duty nursing. Many others were at home caring for their families.

The school was affiliated with the Northwestern University Medical School, met requirements of the National League for Nursing, and annually graduated a class of about 40 students. In 1935, because of Wesley's deficit of $16,515.11 and a lack of jobs open for nurses at hospitals across the country, the school was forced to close temporarily. The Wesley Alumnae

Association helped place the year's graduates at the University of Chicago Hospitals and Clinics and other institutions. The residence where staff nurses lived also was closed and Wesley nurses were housed in the unoccupied patient rooms in the Hospital.

NEW OFFICERS NAMED

George W. Dixon, who had succeeded Perley Lowe as president after his death in July, 1924, was named honorary president, a new office, at the Wesley Board of Trustees meeting in January, 1935. Vice President Frederick John Thielbar, trustee since 1908, was elected president.

Although Dixon's ten-year tenure had spanned the depths of the depression, Wesley had made a number of improvements during its struggle for survival. The annual reports from 1930 through 1935 (mimeographed to save money) showed resurgent interest in repairing and re-equipping the old building as hopes dimmed for moving to the new location. Superintendent Paul H. Fesler reported that new scientific equipment purchased in 1932 included a microtome, projectoscope, gas machine for anesthesia and an electrocardiograph. During the three years following, operating rooms and delivery rooms were repaired and painted, and a new dining room for interns was opened. The steam boilers were overhauled and the laundry, closed for a year, was reopened with new washing machines. New equipment was installed in the diet kitchen and, for the first time, private patients were given a selection of food from menus.

The Hospital was particularly proud of its accomplishments in 1934 when 18 Northwestern Medical School graduates applied for internships at Wesley. Among the 13 young physicians accepted was Theodore R. Van Dellen who would in time join the Passavant staff and become a widely read medical columnist of the *Chicago Tribune*. Superintendent Fesler's report stated, "The Hospital has endeavored to meet every request from the Medical School and from members of the faculty in connection with the teaching program. We now have regular scheduled clinics in all departments, and, from all reports, the officers of the Medical School as well as the clinicians are much interested."

Northwestern Medical School's desire to control Wesley's teaching beds waned when the school's affiliation with Passavant Memorial Hospital[1] was effected in 1925. Northwestern had engaged a new dean, Dr. Irving Samuel Cutter, to develop the medical school on the Chicago campus according to the requirements of Mrs. Montgomery Ward in memorializing her husband. Dr. Cutter considered a hospital essential in carrying out his plans and he guided Passavant in erecting a new building on the southeast corner of Superior Street and Fairbanks Court, diagonally across from Wesley's projected hospital property.

Ground breaking ceremonies for the new Passavant were held on February 6, 1928, and the 200-bed hospital was opened to patients June 10, 1929, at the onset of the depression. The majority of the 14 physicians who left Wesley had joined the reorganized Passavant staff.

Wesley's depleted environment, diminished professional staff, deficient financial resources and isolated location, combined with the indifference of Northwestern Medical School, resulted in an all-time low morale of the venerable institution.

A WELCOME WINDFALL

The first good news of the decade was proclaimed at the Union League Club on Saturday, October 14, 1936, when Wesley President Frederick Thielbar announced that George Herbert Jones, vice president of the Board of Trustees, had given one million dollars to construct a new hospital building on Northwestern's Chicago campus.

A reaction of joy permeated Wesley as trustees called for construction bids and employees planned their new departments. The promised building inspired the Woman's Auxiliary Board to make elaborate plans for fund raising. They revised the membership list and devised means to persuade delinquent members to pay back dues. Membership increased to 477. These absorbing activities continued through the winter and spring until Saturday, June 19, 1937 when ground was broken for the new hospital at Superior Street and Fairbanks Court. The first spadeful of earth was turned by Mr. Jones and the ritual ceremony was conducted by Bishop Ernest Lynn Waldorf.

[1]*Passavant Memorial Hospital had been founded in 1865, destroyed by fire in 1871, rebuilt in 1884 and closed in 1925 because of obsolete facilities. Vernon K. Brown, "The Story of Passavant Memorial Hospital."*

104

In the fall of 1937, Paul H. Fesler, superintendent since 1931, announced his resignation. Ernest R. Snyder was appointed acting superintendent.

The Wind Changes

The man who had led Wesley safely through ten of the darkest years, *George William Dixon*, president from 1924 to 1934, died September 8, 1938 at the age of 72. Family and friends were consoled that his last days were brightened by the thought that his greatest desire, Wesley's new building, was assured. Two of Dixon's brothers, Homer Lains Dixon and William Warren Dixon, were serving on the board at the time.

Dr. Allen Buckner Kanavel, eminent surgeon and teacher on the Wesley Staff for 32 years, died May 27, 1938, at the age of 64. Dr. Kanavel had been chairman of Northwestern's department of surgery (1919-1929) and co-editor of the school's Quarterly Bulletin (1907-1912) with his Wesley colleague, *Dr. Charles A. Elliott*, chairman of the department of medicine (1919-1929). Dr. Elliott died June 26, 1939, at the age of 66. Both men had become emeritus at Wesley prior to their deaths. The Wesley medical staff had been further depleted in 1936 through the deaths of *Drs. Payson LaVern Nusbaum, Aloysius James Larkin* and *Otis Hardy Maclay; Dr. Charles B. Younger* had died in 1934; *Drs. Albert B. Yudelson* and *Robert Blue* died in 1939. Deaths among trustees were *Henry Gottlieb Eckstein* and *William Lees*, 1934; *George Dayton Webb*, 1936.

Widespread Darkness

The thirtieth decade ended on the somber note that had ushered it in. Bad weather and uncertain finances brought Wesley's new building to a halt soon after the foundation and sub-structure were completed. The discouraged Hospital repaired and reopened the third floor of the old building to care for an increase in patients.

Nationally, war clouds prevailed even though the United States had proclaimed its neutrality in World War II. German troops marched on Poland September 1, 1939, and France and Great Britain declared war on Germany.

A New Era
1940 to 1960

Part III

The Builders   Chapter 15

Wesley's new building had been dormant for almost three years when construction resumed early in April, 1940. George Herbert Jones had increased his 1936 gift of one million dollars by $500,000 the following year and, in 1940, he added $1,500,000 to assure completion. Sharing as donor with Mr. Jones was his daughter, Mrs. Ruth Jones Jarratt, a Wesley trustee.

Wesley President Frederick John Thielbar presided before a distinguished assemblage at the cornerstone laying May 26, 1940. The Reverend Ernest Lynn Waldorf, resident bishop of the Methodist Church and member of Wesley's executive committee, conducted the ceremony. Dr. Franklin Bliss Snyder, president of Northwestern University and a Wesley trustee, delivered the principal address; Dr. Raymond W. McNealy, chief of Wesley's medical staff, responded; and the man who made the structure possible, George Herbert Jones, spread the mortar to seal the stone in place. Others seated on the platform were the Reverend John Thompson, minister of the Chicago Temple and a Wesley trustee; the Reverend John H. DeLacy, hospital chaplain; M. Haddon MacLean, Wesley treasurer; Kenneth F. Burgess, president of the Northwestern University Board of Trustees; James S. Kemper and Thomas A. Harwood, Wesley trustees.

MEANING OF THE CORNERSTONE

In his introductory remarks, Frederick Thielbar said that "in modern construction, the cornerstone no longer functions in a structural sense, but as a symbol it retains its traditional significance and spiritual meaning." The statement was authentic for Thielbar not only was Wesley's president, but also its architect. He had designed the 20-story building in the form of the letter X, reminiscent of cathedrals of the middle ages. It was he who had drawn the two-story lobby with vaulted ceilings and Gothic pillars; and it was he who first called the building a "Cathedral of Healing."

SUCCESSFUL TOPPING-OFF

During the summer months, construction progressed rapidly and the topping-off ceremony took place in the afternoon of November 15, 1940, before another inportant group of hospital officers and friends. The event was further celebrated by the Woman's Auxiliary Board which sponsored a benefit concert by John Charles Thomas at Orchestra Hall in the evening. The world-famed baritone was a particularly popular choice. As the son of a Methodist minister, John Charles first sang in public at camp meetings where his father preached. His performance brought wide publicity for the new building and $600 toward furnishing a patient room.

TWO GREAT ACHIEVERS FAIL TO SEE COMPLETION

The topping-off was the last building-related ceremony to be attended by two of the new structure's foremost sustainers. The first was George Herbert Jones, trustee since 1924, whose gifts totaling three million dollars made possible the erection of the building. He died suddenly on July 6, 1941, at the age of 85. Jones had been born in Bristol, England, and educated in British schools. At the age of 15 he accompanied his father to Chicago where they settled shortly before the fire of 1871. The young man was employed as a clerk for a firm of iron merchants, Hall, Kimbark & Company, and later became sales manager. In 1893 he helped organize Inland Steel Company and served as the company's second president for eight years. He was known for his achievements in the industrial world and for his philanthropies, especially those related to the Methodist Church, where he had been a lifelong member. In deep appreciation for his màgnanimous gift, the Wesley property was designated the "George Herbert Jones Hospital Center."

The second man who did not live to see his dream materialize was Frederick John Thielbar, who became ill in August and was confined in old Wesley until his death November 15, 1941 at the age of 75. Thielbar had been an architect in Chicago for 49 years and was recognized as an outstanding leader in his profession. He had designed the 22-story Chicago Temple (First Methodist Church), completed in 1924. The spire, rising 568 feet above the tower, was said to be the tallest church spire in the world. In addition to Wesley, Thielbar was a trustee of Northwestern University, Methodist Old People's Home, and Goodwill Industries, and was an active member of the Methodist Church. Long before 1935 when he became Wesley's president, Thielbar, with his partner, John R. Fugard, had considered the structure which would have to go upward to accommodate more than 500 beds in a limited city area. Death came to the master architect exactly one year after the topping-off and three weeks before the dedication of the beautiful building.

THE CATHEDRAL OF HEALING

The new building was formally dedicated Sunday, November 30, 1941. The ceremony took place beneath the gold leaf mural[1], *The Divine Healer*, by John H. DeRosen, noted church artist, in the cathedral-type lobby with marble floors and walls. The dedication address was delivered by the Reverend Ernest Fremont Tittle, minister of the First Methodist Church of Evanston, with Dr. Raymond W. McNealy, Wesley trustee and acting superintendent during the transition period, presiding. Bishop Ernest Lynn Waldorf conducted the ceremony. Approximately 500 persons attended and many more heard the service, which was broadcast over radio station WIND.

The opening week activities continued through Friday, December 5, 1941, when the new Wesley's first patient, Mrs. Minnie K. Weissenbach, was brought by ambulance from old Wesley through the honor guard at the

[1]*The mural illustrated that healing power protected all people throughout the ages. Jesus at the pool of Siloam (John 9.7, Holy Bible) is shown surrounded by 8 widely different types of people. At left is a disciple and a woman holding a baby. At right is an elderly woman, a modern medical student, an injured man supported by a steel worker identified by his heavy apron, and a blind woman.*

front entrance formed by a Red Cross Nurses' Aide Corps at 8:30 p.m. A crowd of spectators (estimated by police at 20,000) filled the foyer and reception room, and stood outside in a line two blocks long waiting to attend the public housewarming and tour the building. Governor of Illinois Dwight H. Green and Mrs. Green headed the welcoming committee at the elevator to greet the patient. Thus, almost 53 years since the three-bed Wesley Hospital admitted Mrs. Hattie Dewar on Christmas Day, 1888, the 535-bed Wesley Memorial Hospital admitted another first patient, beginning a new era in a larger building and with the capacity to deliver much more sophisticated care.

Wesley's imposing edifice continued the classic architectural style of other buildings on Northwestern University's Chicago campus. The exterior walls of the 17-story building plus three-story tower were of white Bedford stone covering the reinforced concrete frame. The decorative motives were largely Gothic but "the architects made no sacrifice of light and air, built up no useless masses of masonry in order to achieve archeological correctness."[1]

The entrance opened to a two-story lobby with pillars, arches and vaulted ceilings. Though the building form and lobby harked back to medieval cathedrals, there the resemblance ended. This building embraced the most modern arrangements, materials and equipment then known for medical treatment, safety and comfort of patients.

Plan of Wesley
Memorial Hospital

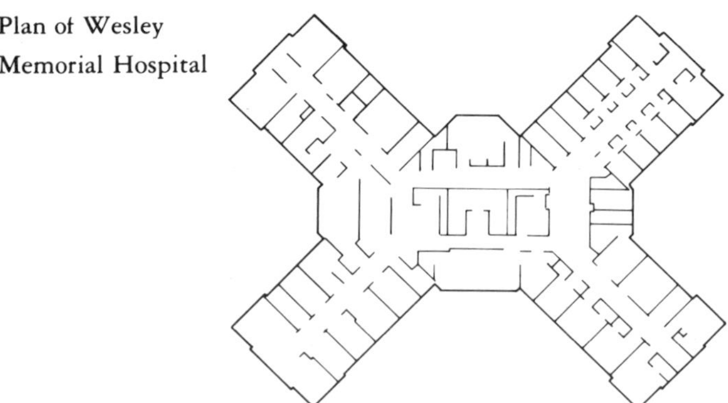

[1]*"New Version of the Vertical Hospital, Wesley Memorial Hospital, Chicago"* Architectural Record. *August, 1944*

The X shape was formed by the double V floor plan where two large Vs with wings at 90 degree angles were joined against the central shaft, the point of each being located at the center. Each of the side elements was a patient floor with the nurses' stations in the central shaft at the point of the letter V, providing excellent nursing control. The V plan guaranteed sunshine in every patient room at some time of day and minimum traffic in corridors. The central shaft, like a tree trunk, functioned as a vertical supply line. Most supplies came up in pneumatic tubes and conveyors of various types. High-speed electrically heated dumbwaiters enabled Wesley to serve meals to 600 patients in less than an hour and a half.

Elevators in the central shaft further controlled traffic. Wards were on the lower floors. The patient population decreased as the floors rose and the rooms became larger and more expensive. The daily rate for most rooms was seven or eight dollars, although quarters on the topmost floors could reach twenty-five dollars.

The doors to patient rooms were four feet wide to permit patients to be moved in their beds to lounges and solariums on the top floors with splendid views of Lake Michigan. On the 17th floor, the roofs of the four wings of the Vs were floored with wood plank over asphalt, and the plumbing vent pipes were covered and arranged to form a frame for a canvas marquee.

YULE CELEBRATIONS OF ALL NATIONS
During opening week the Woman's Auxiliary Board took full advantage of the 18th floor solarium, an octagon of solid glass windows affording a panorama of Chicago. Members presented a two-day Christmas Fiesta for visitors. International booths were staffed by girls in native dress offering handcrafts, toys and exotic delicacies, which netted three thousand dollars for the Hospital. On both days nurses' aides in pale blue uniforms and white Dutch caps guided more than a thousand visitors through the building. They saw patients' rooms with two-way speaking systems and soundproof ceilings, the pediatric floor with decorated playrooms, the physical therapy department with gymnasium and swimming pool and the surgical floor with every scientific device then known to aid the surgeon.

Women, especially, were amazed at a kitchen with its own bakery, salad room, meat shop and ice cream plant, each in self-contained units, a kitchen capable of processing 4,500 pounds of raw food and preparing 3,500 meals each day.

First Nursery Occupants Arrive

Guests viewed the obstetrical floor with three large labor rooms and five delivery rooms equipped for improved scientific procedures to safeguard the mother and her newborn. The nursery had 40 bassinets and, of course, the "Stork Club" for expectant fathers.

The nursery was activated on Tuesday, December 9, when its first occupant, John Wesley Engels, was born to Mr. and Mrs. Frank A. Engels, at 3:41 a.m. The new Wesley's first baby, named for the religious leader for whom old Wesley Hospital was named, was joined in the nursery at 1:24 p.m. on the same day, December 9, by Susanna Wesley Grabske. She was the first baby girl born in the new hospital and was named for the mother of John Wesley. The infant's parents were Mr. and Mrs. William Grabske. Hence a tradition that began March 18, 1889, was continued when the first baby in Chicago's old Wesley Hospital was named Susanna Wesley Lentz. This had been a quick switch in the plans of parents and deaconess nurses who had hoped for a boy to bear the name of John Wesley himself.

After a tour through the building, Robert M. Yoder wrote a descriptive article[1] asserting:

> "The first instrument ever used in this $4,000,000 hospital was a light meter such as photographers use to determine the exposure. Engineers went in as soon as the plaster was dry, measuring the amount and kind of light in every room. The first prescription written was for color—color in every room, compounded as carefully as an order of medicine.
>
> "White went into the discard—the only white in this hospital is the nurses' uniforms and the mashed potatoes. Also discarded was that favorite shade of public-building interiors, sweet potato tan. Instead, rooms with northern exposure are decorated in warm shades of coral and lemon yellow, rooms to the south with cool shades of aquamarine and what the experts call pale sea-foam green. In the wards, which use the same color scheme as the most expensive private room in the house, you find beds enameled coral or turquoise, walls tinted yellow or pale green.

[1]*Robert M. Yoder "Let's be Sick in Comfort," Saturday Evening Post, July 10, 1943.*

"There are none of the white iron bedsteads of old-fashioned hospitals, and none of the sanitary-looking metal furniture with imitation wood finishes. This furniture is period stuff in mahogany or maple, exactly like that found in a good hotel or club. On the sixteenth floor, before it was taken over for the use of Navy men in and around Chicago, they used Chinese Chippendale furniture and Chinese prints. Only the extra height of the beds—thirty-four inches to the top of the mattress—indicates that this is a hospital."

DAYS OF OPPORTUNITY—AND DESTINY

On Sunday, December 7, 1941, with the opening fanfare over and the patients safe in their rooms, Wesley quietly turned to its expanded responsibility for caring for the sick and teaching young physicians.

Ironically, this was the same day that the Japanese naval and air forces made their infamous attack on the United States Pacific fleet at Pearl Harbor and our country again was committed to world warfare.

Following the unexpected death of Frederick Thielbar, on November 15, Thomas J. Thomas was named president of Wesley. However, he was called to Washington on a patriotic mission and resigned a few months after taking office. At a meeting of the Board of Trustees on March 25, 1942, John Holmes, a new member, was elected president. George W. Dixon, Jr., attorney with Sims, Handy and McKnight, whose father had served as president for ten years, was named vice president. Jay L. Hench, president of the Midwest Forging and Manufacturing Company, became treasurer.

Holmes had accompanied his parents from Belfast, Ireland, to the United States in 1891, when he was six years old. At age 15 he was employed as a messenger boy for Swift & Company, became president in 1937 and was chairman of its board, 1955-1959.

In Wesley's Annual Report of 1942, Holmes emphasized the necessity for business efficiency in order to provide service:

"...It would seem to have been almost an act of Providence that our new building was completed and fully equipped at the time it was. Had there been even a three months' delay, it would have been next to impossible to have obtained the necessary equipment, and consequently Wesley would not have been able to take its place of enlarged service...We want all friends of Wesley to know that while of necessity much emphasis has been placed during the year upon improving the business efficiency of the Hospital, it has been with the sole aim of making Wesley a better instrument of service in the healing of the sick. Your officers keep constantly in mind that business efficiency in Wesley is not an end in itself, but a means to an end, that of justifying the term, 'Cathedral of Healing.'

"During the year we were successful in renting our old premises to the Board of Health of the City of Chicago for operation as an Intensive Treatment Center. Thus Old Wesley continues under a new name and administration in its role as a place of healing. Renting this property relieves us of upkeep and provides some non-operating revenue...Wesley desires to maintain cordial relationships with other hospitals and agencies interested in the sick. We are gratified, therefore, that Wesley has been admitted to membership in the Chicago Hospital Council which provides a vehicle for cooperation in improving the operation of member hospitals."

WASHINGTON BOULEVARD STAFF JOINS WESLEY

Although Wesley moved to the new building with only 40 active medical staff members, the group increased to 106 within a year. This remarkable growth was due in large part to the efforts of Dr. Raymond W. McNealy and his successor as chief of staff, Dr. Gilbert H. Marquardt, with the full cooperation of Dr. J. Roscoe Miller who had been appointed dean of the medical school after the retirement of Dr. Irving S. Cutter in May, 1941. The new staff members received appointments to the Northwestern faculty.

The Washington Boulevard Hospital provided an opportune source of high-caliber physicians and nurses. After 30 years of operation in a gradually declining West Side environment and the closure in 1941 of Rush Medical College with which the hospital was associated, its service was terminated on June 30, 1942. The hospital was founded in 1913 by Dr. Albert I. Bouffleur, chief surgeon of the Chicago, Milwaukee, St. Paul and Pacific Railroad; his associate, Dr. Arthur R. Metz; and Dr. B. Franklin Lounsbury who, with a group of medical friends, formed the original staff.

Half of the staff of 18 physicians joined the Wesley staff and Northwestern University faculty July 1, 1942, and the others were appointed to the Hospital's courtesy group. The new Wesley staff members were Dr. Arthur R. Metz, president of the Washington Boulevard Hospital; Dr. Vincent J. O'Conor, vice president; Dr. James F. DePree, Dr. Raymond Householder,

Dr. Robert L. Ladd, Dr. Linn F. McBride, Dr. H. Ivan Sippy, Dr. J. Kenneth Sokol, and Dr. Virgil Wescott.

The following became members of the courtesy group: Dr. James F. Cox, Dr. George G. Hallenbeck, Dr. George McAuliff, Dr. Joseph Prendergast, Dr. T. G. Remmert, Dr. Robert Snively, Dr. Frederick Tice, Dr. Paul Van Verst, and Dr. Harry O. Wernicke.

School of Nursing Reopens

An additional benefit from the Washington Boulevard Hospital alliance was its class of 48 student nurses who, in July, 1942, became the first class in the reopened Wesley Memorial Hospital School of Nursing. Sixty new students were enrolled September 14 and the revived school was off to a healthy start. All students met the requirements of Northwestern University, with which the school was affiliated.

The problem of housing students was solved when Wesley acquired the 17-story Hampshire House at 202 East Delaware Place as a residence for student nurses. The large, attractive apartment building, purchased for $457,500, was remodeled to include nursing arts laboratories and classrooms as well as living quarters. Basic sciences and other courses were taught by Wesley physicians who also were Northwestern faculty members. The students gained clinical experience through assignments at the Hospital and the Montgomery Ward Clinics at the Medical School.

At graduation exercises in the spring of 1945, 43 students, the first Wesley graduates in ten years, received diplomas in nursing. They were honored at a banquet attended by Mae Belle Kellogg (Class of 1892), oldest living Wesley alumnae, and members of the Classes of 1900, 1905 and 1910. In September of the same year, 48 more students were graduated, adding 91 new nurses with Wesley diplomas, the majority remaining in nursing service in the Hospital.

Miss Knapp Retires After 35 Years

Bertha L. Knapp, director of Wesley's School of Nursing and Nursing Service, announced her retirement on September 1, 1943, the 35th anniversary of her appointment to Wesley. A graduate of the University of Michigan School of Nursing, she had served as assistant superintendent of nursing at her alma mater and later as supervisor of the Visiting Nurse

Association of Chicago. She was one of the first nurses appointed by the Governor of Illinois to the State Board of Nurse Examiners and she held many offices in state and regional nursing organizations. Wesley's Board of Directors conferred on Miss Knapp emeritus status for exceptional service to the Hospital and the nursing profession.

During Miss Knapp's tenure more than 1,000 nurses were graduated from Wesley even though the school was closed for eight years. Among the graduates holding important positions elsewhere were Frances Wilson, superintendent of Cheelo University Hospital, Tsinan, China; Maggie Kay Prentice, Isabelle Fisher Hospital, Tientsin, China; Caroline M. Fenby, Superintendent of Methodist Hospital, Madison, Wisconsin; Margaret Johnston, superintendent of Beloit Municipal Hospital, Wisconsin; Faith Serrill, superintendent of Lincoln General Hospital, Nebraska; Mary K. West, superintendent of Methodist Hospital of Southern California, Los Angeles; Sena H. Brandt, superintendent of nurses, Broadlawns Hospital, Des Moines, Iowa; Ada Belle McCleery, superintendent of Evanston Hospital, Illinois, for 20 years; Kathryn Powell, director of Men's Health Service, Northwestern University, Evanston; Mary Bogardus, director of nursing service, University of Chicago Clinics; Eleanor Wilson, nurse in charge of Dental Clinics, Northwestern University Dental School, Chicago; Nell Millard, instructor in sciences, School of Nursing, Michael Reese Hospital, Chicago; Dr. Charlotte Gregory, practicing obstetrician in Chicago.

A 1928 Wesley graduate, Martha Johnson[1], spent 46 years in a nursing career of constant challenge and growth. She earned a master's degree in public health at Johns Hopkins University, Baltimore, where she later became assistant director of the outpatient department. She returned to Chicago and was appointed supervisor of Northwestern University Clinics, then went to New York as head nurse of the outpatient department of New York Hospital—Cornell Medical Center. Later, she was assistant to Kenneth Babcock, M.D., director of the Joint Commission on Accreditation of Hospitals until 1961, when she became director of the Division of Nursing of the American Hospital Association. Miss Johnson remained in this position, one of the nation's top nursing posts, until her retirement in 1974.

---

[1]*"Wesley Life", 1966*

Daughter of Deaconess Nurse Heads New School

Harriet H. Smith, former associate professor of nursing at the University of Washington and director of the School of Nursing and nursing service at Harborview Hospital in Seattle, was named Wesley's superintendent of nurses and director of the school, effective January 1, 1944. Miss Smith was the daughter of a physician and a nurse, her appointment creating an interesting coincidence: her mother had served as supervisor of the deaconess nurses when Wesley Hospital was organized in 1888.

Harriet Smith's experience had been broad and varied. She had taught home nursing in a Red Cross Hospital at Mt. Vernon, Washington; had been nursing supervisor at the Hunan-Yale Hospital in Changsha, China, and had served in the same capacity at New Haven Hospital, New Haven, Connecticut.

Penicillin Research

In the early days of the war, Wesley doctors were conducting research on the new therapeutic agent, penicillin, discovered in 1941. Its use was confined to the armed forces until 1943, when large-scale production made possible a limited supply for civilian use. Wesley had a monthly allotment of "thirty million units of this valuable substance which is proving so efficacious in the treatment of those conditions for which it is indicated. Certain members of the Wesley staff are constantly at work on research problems concerning the further use of penicillin."[1]

Among the investigations assigned to the new residents under the direction of physicians on the medical staff were:

- Penicillin in subacute bacterial endocarditis.
- Penicillin inhalation in respiratory disease.
- Effect of penicillin on the complications of, and termination of, the carrier state in scarlet fever as opposed to other methods of therapy.
- Influenza experimental meningitis. Comparison in various types of therapy.

Deaths on the Home Front

The war-torn first half of the decade brought a number of deaths unrelated to the war.

[1]*Annual Report of Wesley Memorial Hospital, 1944*

The *Reverend Ernest Lynn Waldorf*, Methodist resident bishop in Chicago for 13 years and a member of the Wesley Board of Trustees, died July 27, 1943. Bishop Waldorf had participated with warm and genial guidance during the building opening ceremonies and the trying period of war.

William W. Dixon, member of the Board of Trustees who served as its legal advisor, died December 4, 1940. His valuable counsel guided the trustees through several critical periods.

Dr. Charles Bert Reed, member of the Wesley medical staff for 35 years, died September 3, 1940. He was head of the department of obstetrics for 28 years and served as chief of staff for three terms.

Dr. William Miller, surgeon, who had been elected chief of the Wesley medical staff on January 18, 1941, died on the following February 22. After completing his internship at Wesley in 1912, he joined the Northwestern University faculty and the Wesley medical staff where he served for 30 years.

Wesley and World War II — Chapter 16

ctivating a new hospital building while adjusting to a wartime economy presented challenges rarely met in the hospital field. At its former location Wesley patients had dropped to an average of 90 by 1941 and its medical, nursing and operating staffs had decreased accordingly. In its new home with a potential of 600 beds, Wesley had to cope with priorities, food rationing, scarcity of supplies and personnel losses to the armed forces and industry, while simultaneously recruiting both professional and operational personnel. The Hospital had to be staffed before wartime obligations or civilian needs could be fulfilled.

Dr. Raymond W. McNealy, Wesley's chief of staff, had temporarily suspended a busy surgical practice in 1940 to serve as superintendent during the Hospital's transition period. His leadership facilitated the move from Chicago's south side to the near north side with a minimum of disruption. Dr. McNealy resigned February 1, 1942 to resume his practice and Edgar Blake, Jr., his assistant, assumed administrative duties. Blake was a graduate of Wesleyan University at Middletown, Connecticut, and had served as superintendent of the Methodist Hospital of Gary, Indiana.

The nucleus of personnel was formed by department heads from Old Wesley including Bertha L. Knapp (retired in 1943), nursing service; Emma L. Grimm, acting director, nursing education; Dr. Frank L. Hussey, radiologist; Dr. Emory R. Strauser, pathologist; Dr. Mary Karp, anesthesiologist; Adelaide Venetucci, chief pharmacist; Elizabeth L. Tuft, executive dietitian, and Otto G. Bodemer, purchasing agent. Among the new employees heading departments were Joseph L. Williams, assistant superintendent, from Columbia Hospital in Milwaukee; Joseph L. Champley, chief engineer; and Hertha P. McCully, executive housekeeper, from corresponding positions at the Lake Shore Drive Hotel. When the army took over the Stevens Hotel (now the Conrad Hilton), its accountant, Herbert C. Jensen, and credit manager, Charles F. Street, came to Wesley to fill the same positions. Other new administrative personnel were Alice A. Chesbrown, chief physical therapist; Katherine N. Williams, medical social worker; Charles S. Watson, personnel director; and Kathryn S. Walsh, director of volunteer services. Edna K. Huffman, medical records librarian, was a president of the American Association of Medical Record Librarians before joining Wesley.

DOCTORS JOIN ARMED FORCES, STAFF REORGANIZED
Thirty-one members of the medical staff already had joined the armed forces by 1942 including Chief of Staff Gilbert H. Marquardt, who was succeeded by Dr. Gerard N. Krost. The staff was reorganized with new bylaws providing a larger and more representative executive committee. In his report for 1942, Dr. Krost stressed the teaching activities of the staff.

"A prerequisite for membership on the staff is being a member of the faculty of Northwestern University Medical School...The hospital facilities are being used for teaching to an even greater degree. We have assigned to the Hospital senior medical students who serve as student clerks and who, through the divisions of medicine, surgery and obstetrics, come in direct contact with the patients by writing histories, examining the patients and following the course of their condition. A new clinical meeting called *Grand Rounds* is conducted by medical residents each Monday morning...The student clerks and interns discuss freely the various aspects of the diagnosis and treatment of the more interesting types of cases. Thus the residents receive experience in teaching and the student clerks learn by making individual observations unhampered by the ordinary pedagogic approach...Five classes are conducted in the Hospital by members of the staff...Numerous members have regular classes and dispensary work in the Medical School. We also give lectures to the pupils in the School of Nursing."

Before Wesley's two top floors with solariums could be used by civilian patients, the Navy requested them as a hospital facility for sick men at Navy Pier. The majority were trainees in the V7 Naval Reserve Midshipmen's Unit who lived in the university's new dormitory, Abbott Hall. Specialty Naval Unit No. 29 provided the medical and nursing care for a daily average of 200 Navy enlisted personnel at Wesley throughout the war. The Hospital provided x-ray and laboratory work required in examination of inductees for the Army Induction Center. Wives of Army and Navy men were given medical service when needed.

TRAINING FOR OVERSEAS

Another branch of Wesley's war service was the intensive preparation of young men and women for medical and nursing service in the armed forces.

The *Medical Education Program* began in March, 1943. Each quarter during the war, 20 to 25 students from the Northwestern Medical School senior class were assigned to Wesley as clerk participants in a nine-month internship which would normally take 12 months. The clerkships familiarized them with patients' histories, laboratories and other units within the Hospital. After intensive training under residents' supervision, they were commissioned directly into the United States Army, Navy, Marines or Public Health Service.

The *United States Cadet Nurse Corps* was an accelerated program starting in July, 1943, to prepare young women for service in the armed forces or the home front. Wesley enrolled 172 cadets who attended lectures by medical faculty members and nursing classes taught by nurse supervisors of medical, operating room, obstetric and pediatric services. Wesley received $169,229.06 to support participation in the United States Cadet Nurse program authorized by Congress.

WARTIME NURSE RECRUITMENT SCENE

Wesley was the setting and provided the cast for a motion picture, *"R.N.—Serving All Mankind"* produced by the American College of Surgeons under a grant from the Becton Dickinson Foundation. Wesley nurses and interns acted their real life roles before cameras in the emergency department, nursery, surgical suite, laboratories and private rooms. The film was made in response to the Surgeon General's request for 55,000 students to enter accredited nursing schools in the fall of 1942. The Chicago premiere was held in the Murphy Memorial Auditorium and later was shown throughout the country.

VOLUNTEERS FOR VICTORY

A report of Wesley volunteers must begin with the *Woman's Auxiliary Board*, which started in 1889 as the Ladies Aid Association to help the struggling young hospital. Over the years they tirelessly sewed gowns, layettes and hospital linens. They collected food from farms and neighbors, rolled bandages and increased in numbers and competence. As Wesley grew, their activities expanded to sponsoring imaginative events which earned substantial sums to furnish wards, provide children's hospital care, and buy essential equipment; and they served with fortitude in World War I. By 1943, membership had grown to 787, a large group of devoted women helping wherever needed in the dark days of World War II.

The *Susanna Wesley Circle* was organized by the Auxiliary Board members' daughters and young friends who first called themselves the Junior Auxiliary. This initial group became inactive, but in 1943 they reorganized and changed the name to honor Susanna Wesley, mother of John Wesley, for whom the Hospital was named. In its first year the group furnished a patient room, made hundreds of Christmas toys for pediatric patients and stuffed Christmas stockings for patients on the navy floors.

The *Wesley Service Club* was started in 1935 by wives and friends of staff physicians. Its members established and devoted their full attention to the Wesley Gift Shop, keeping it as well stocked as possible during the wartime merchandise shortage. Proceeds went to the pediatric unit.

In addition to Wesley's women's groups, the Hospital was assisted by agencies and individuals who responded to national appeals for workers in hospitals serving both war and home needs on skeletal staffs. The *American Red Cross* assigned to Wesley members of its *Nurse Aide Corps* who had completed 80 hours of training. These women gave baths and bedside care, and performed kindly tasks for patients, freeing nurses for duties requiring professional training. *Red Cross Gray Ladies* filled in at nursing stations, reception desks and countless vacancies. One of Wesley's 163 Gray Ladies, Mrs. Ruth Jones Jarett, was a co-donor of the new building with her father, George Herbert Jones. She also donated the patients' library and frequently staffed the book cart which was circulated daily to all patients. Members of the *Red Cross Canteen Service* worked in the kitchen with dietary personnel. They helped arrange trays on the conveyor belt and passed trays to patients on the floors.

The American Women's Voluntary Services was organized in 1943 specifically for supplementary typing, filing and other office services. These volunteers worked in the pharmacy, laboratories, central supply and administrative offices. Many were career women who gave their evenings when the employee shortage was critical.

The *Victory Volunteers* began in 1943 to provide extensive service, especially in the evenings and on Sundays, performing whatever tasks needed to be done.

Members of the different *Methodist Church Auxiliaries* in metropolitan Chicago gave one day a week rolling bandages, making dressings and assembling supplies for the obstetrical department.

The *Jangos* (Junior Army and Navy Guild Organization) were the daughters, wives and sisters of Army and Navy officers. In red, white and blue uniforms, they served on the Navy floors, assisted in the service shop and staffed the shop cart.

The *Men's Volunteer Corps* also was organized in 1943 to assist nurses in the operating rooms and the men's wards, as well as to help the oxygen technicians.

The total number of volunteer hours at Wesley in 1943 amounted to the incredible sum of 63,396 divided among the groups as follows: Red Cross Nurses Aides, 17,378; Red Cross Gray Ladies, 20,779; Red Cross Canteen Workers, 1,627; A.W.V.S., 10,409; Victory Volunteers, 8,022; Methodist Church Women's groups (9 months), 3,762; Jangos (3 months), 1,340; Men's Volunteer Corps (1 month), 79. During the five war years, 1941 through 1946, Red Cross volunteers and those of other agencies gave 260,000 hours of service to Wesley.

The title "Victory Volunteers," was selected by one group, but actually applied to all the unaffiliated individuals who answered the call for help as a patriotic service. The entire volunteer program was coordinated by Kathryn S. Walsh, supervisor of Volunteer Services who had worked in the same capacity at the University of Michigan Hospital at Ann Arbor.

Without the strength and dependability of its volunteers, Wesley's service doubtless would have been seriously curtailed during World War II. Superintendent Edgar Blake, Jr., said "Many hospitals would have had to close their doors were it not for the Victory Volunteers."

Hospitals continued to benefit from volunteer service which began as patriotism. Many persons who had experienced the satisfaction of helping others continued to serve when the pressures of war had ceased. Their intelligence, strength and high motivation have added a quality to hospital care that no amount of money could buy.

REPORTS FROM THE WAR ZONE

From 1942 through 1945, doctors and nurses at Wesley received letters from colleagues stationed from England to New Guinea and Guadalcanal as well as from various parts of the United States. *Lt. Col. Gilbert H. Marquardt*, former Wesley chief of staff, in charge of the U.S. Army Air Corps Department at Coral Gables, Florida, known as Stationary Hospital No. 1, wrote that he had returned from an overseas inspection trip covering 21,000 miles.

Commander J. Roscoe Miller, M.C., U.S.N.R., dean of Northwestern University Medical School and member of Wesley's Board of Directors and medical staff, was appointed Chief of the Section of Medicine, Professional Division, Bureau of Medicine and Surgery, U.S.N. in Washington, D.C. His duties were to investigate medical departments of the U.S. Naval Hospitals and make recommendations.

Among the Wesley physicians and nurses stationed in England were *Maj. Felix Jansey*, M.C., U.S.A.; *Maj. William A. Loeppert*, flight surgeon; *Lts. Jewel Summers* and *Lydia Ghiring*, both Nurse Corps, U.S.A., who wrote of their work in a hospital in England. *Lt. Clemetta Spanier*, Nurse Corps, U.S.A., reported that she was a patient in England after assignment to an air evacuation squadron in France. From France came word that *Lt. Col. Hampar Kelikian* and *Lt. Ian Chesser* happened to meet while on duty.

Maj. J. Fred Merritt spent two years in North Africa and Italy as a base surgeon in the Army Air Corps before returning to Randolph Field, Texas. Serving in the China-Burma-India theater were *Lts. Dorothy Schulz* and *Betty Steenbergen* who were assigned to a unit of the 20th General Hospital.

Wesley nurses with the 12th General Hospital, the Northwestern University Unit, *Sylvia Augspurger, Elsie Buran* and *Elizabeth Boyd*, wrote that they were traveling during the third consecutive Christmas but were still stationed in Italy. *Lt. Eleanor McNamara*, first Wesley nurse to enter the service, was based in a hospital in Italy.

U.S. NAVY IN THE SOUTH PACIFIC
Lt. Comdr. Philip Shambaugh, M.C., U.S.N.R., wrote in May, 1945, that he was in his 11th month of overseas duty aboard the battleship USS North Carolina, had participated in action in Leyte, Luzon, Iwo Jima, Okinawa and was becoming battle-weary.

Lt. Comdr. James K. Stack spent a seven-day leave in Chicago wearing the Philippine Liberation Medal and the Unit Citation given the Fifth Fleet for its part in the invasion of Okinawa. He was assigned to the USS Tazewell.

A note from *Lt. Comdr. Donald K. Hibbs*, M.C., U.S.N.R., postmarked Iwo Jima, dated March 17, 1945, thanked *Emma L. Grimm*, assistant nursing service director and editorial board member of a new publication, *The Wesley Commentator*, sent to all Wesley people overseas. He wrote in part, "This is the first news I have had of Wesley since leaving last July and the picture on the cover (Wesley on NUMS campus) was a sight for sore eyes. The island is secured now so we may see civilization for a while as the 5th Amphibious Corps is reformed..."

The Wesley Commentator brought another response from *Lt. Comdr. John M. Bailey* who was with the Medical Government Section in the Pacific. He said he was at Base Hospital No. 8 but soon would return "to the work in which I can make the greatest contribution (Military Government) to help end the war."

Lt. Norman C. Meyer, M.C., U.S.N.R. assigned to the USS Butte, had a 12-day leave in Chicago before returning to the South Pacific. *Lt. Comdr. Herman Chor*, M.C., U.S.N.R., wrote from Mare Island that he had spent 21 months as head of the department of neuro-psychiatry in a naval base hospital.

ARMY ACTION IN THE SOUTH PACIFIC
Lt. Col. H. Ivan Sippy, M.C., U.S.A., who came to Wesley from the Washington Boulevard Hospital, was chief of the cardiovascular department of the 13th General Hospital (derived from Rush Medical College and its associated teaching hospitals) at their stations in the United States,

Australia and New Guinea. In 1944 he was transferred and became Commanding Officer of the 248th General Hospital, which moved from New Guinea to Luzon and was made part of the 26th Hospital Center. After the Japanese surrender, Colonel Sippy contracted a series of near-fatal illnesses and was returned by hospital ship to the United States in November, 1945.

Colonel Sippy told of a friend, *Charles A. Stafford,* a Washington Boulevard intern at the time of the merger, who had joined the Army Air Force early in the war. As a medical officer in the Southwest Pacific theater, he was conducting a group of patients in an attempted air evacuation from Java when they were shot down by a Japanese attack plane, with total annihilation. As a tribute to the heroic doctor, a hospital ship that served in that theater during the rest of World War II was named "The Stafford."

Lt. Soledad Huerta, a Washington Boulevard graduate who joined Wesley's nursing service, served in the Army Nurse Corps, first in Australia and then in Luzon where she hoped to meet her brother, a prisoner of the Japanese. *Lt. Mildred Greider*, assistant in the Wesley nursing service before entering the service in 1942, was stationed in New Caledonia. *Capt. Mildred Mulliken* wrote from somewhere in the South Pacific that her brother was in charge of a hospital at New Guinea and that one of his nurses, *Lt. Florence Finger*, was her classmate at Wesley (Class of 1931).

Even before Japan's surrender came good news for Wesley. *Lt. Eleanor Garen* (Class of 1931), Army Nurse Corps, who had volunteered for service in January, 1941, was liberated from Santo Tomas Prison Camp in Manila. She had been assigned to Fort Benning, Georgia, then sent to the Philippines, on to Corregidor, then to Bataan. She returned to Corregidor, which was surrendered to the Japanese May 6, 1942. In July, Lieutenant Garen and 66 other nurses were interned in Santo Tomas Prison Camp. She remained there until U.S. Army units liberated the internees February 3, 1945, then was flown to her home in South Bend, Indiana. Her service decorations included the American Defense Ribbon with 1 Bronze Star, Asiatic-Pacific Theater with 2 Battle Stars, Philippine Defense Ribbon and Bronze Star for duty in Prison Camp.

MORE GOOD NEWS
Maj. Edwin A. Wegner, M.C., 120th General Hospital, U.S.A., wrote from

Manila on June 4, 1945: "I left New Guinea late in January and headed north as ship's surgeon on a Liberty ship. Arrived here too late to see Lt. Eleanor Garen. We have taken over right where she left off.

"We have a large hospital serving as an evacuation hospital until this area quiets down. Surgery is busy 24 hours a day with four surgical teams alternating on time. The operating rooms are screened and located in permanent buildings. In this way men are flown in or come by ambulance, some as soon as one and one half hours after injury.

"It looks like the Philippines will be a big hospital center for future army activities north and west of here. Greetings to everyone and I hope I can get back to work with you by Christmas." Major Wegner was prophetic, for Japan surrendered September 2, 1945, making it possible for him and many Wesley colleagues to be home or en route by Christmas.

SERVICE MEN AND WOMEN RETURN HOME

With the world at peace once more, medical and nursing staff members returned to Wesley to resume clinical and teaching responsibilities. In anticipation, the Hospital had extended the private staff office area on the second floor, so the veteran doctors could start medical practice immediately rather than wait until they could set up private offices.

Northwestern University Medical School had expanded its postgraduate teaching program which was conducted mostly in Wesley and Passavant, its affiliated teaching hopitals. Wesley assumed its share of the work planned primarily for young physicians from the armed forces who wished specialty training under the G.I. Bill of Rights. Although the Hospital continued to take interns for twelve-month periods, residents were selected from returning veterans only. Twenty-five of the new residents became engaged in research already under way, in addition to their routine duties specified in the residency programs.

According to Wesley records, the names and ranks of Wesley doctors at time of entry in the armed forces, excluding those mentioned, were:

Col. Harry M. Hedge, M.C., U.S.A.
Col. Ralph F. MacDonald, M.C., U.S.A.
Lt. Col. Loyal Davis, M.C., U.S.A.
Lt. Col. Max C. Ehrlich, M.C., U.S.A.
Lt. Col. Earl I. Greene, M.C., U.S.A.

Lt. Col. Byford B. Heskett, M.C., U.S.A.
Lt. Col. William J. Pickett, M.C., U.S.A.
Lt. Col. Leander W. Riba, M.C., U.S.A.
Maj. Benjamin Boshes, M.C., U.S.A.
Maj. Maurice Gore, M.C., U.S.A.
Maj. John E. Karabin, M.C., U.S.A.
Maj. Frederick Lieberthal, M.C., U.S.A.
Maj. John Martin, M.C., U.S.A.
Maj. John H. Mohardt, M.C., U.S.A.
Maj. J. Peerman Nesselrod, M.C., U.S.A.
Maj. Richard A. Perritt, M.C., U.S.A.
Maj. O. Theodore Roberg, M.C., U.S.A.
Maj. Joseph E. Schaefer, M.C., U.S.A.
Maj. Paul L. Shallenberger, M.C., U.S.A.
Maj. Durand Smith, M.C., U.S.A.
Capt. Albert Andrews, M.C., U.S.A.
Capt. Harold Eisenstein, M.C., U.S.A.
Capt. Homer B. Field, M.C., U.S.A.
Capt. Standiford Helm, M.C., U.S.A.
Capt. Milo E. Jeffries, M.C., U.S.A.
Capt. Chester Lockwood, M.C., U.S.A.
Capt. Irving Puntenney, M.C., U.S.A.
Capt. Ralph C. Roberts, M.C., U.S.A.
Capt. Reno P. Rosi, M.C., U.S.A.
Capt. Ching Tai Tong, M.C., U.S.A.
Capt. S. Lloyd Teitelman, M.C., U.S.A.
Lt. James W. Hall, M.C., U.S.A.
Lt. Theodore Van Dellen, M.C., U.S.A.

Capt. Edwin DeCosta, M.C., U.S.N.R.
Lt. Comdr. Leonard DeLozier, M.C., U.S.N.R.
Lt. Comdr. William W. Sittler, M.C., U.S.N.R.
Lt. John A. Gubler, M.C., U.S.N.R.

Converting to Peace   Chapter 17

Although Wesley had occupied its new building five years, operations on an all-civilian basis were reviewed for the first time in its 58th Annual Report covering the fiscal year, September 1, 1945 to August 31, 1946. After restoring two glass-enclosed floors containing navy patient accommodations to their original purpose as patient lounging facilities, Wesley had 560 patient beds and 50 bassinets. Financial data in Superintendent Blake's report revealed that Wesley's assets including land, building, equipment, endowment funds, restricted funds and cash in the bank totaled $7,443,450.98. The James Deering Fund was $1,096,613.12 and the General Free Bed Endowment Fund was $771,241.65, income from which was $39,301.94 (Deering) and $27,048.80 (General Free Bed) representing a return of 3.58 and 3.51 percent on the investment of the respective funds. The income enabled Wesley to give $272,395 of free and part pay care of which patients paid only $40,447. A large proportion of the patients came to the Hospital through the Montgomery Ward Clinics of the Northwestern University Medical School.

Further analysis of Wesley's financial standing showed that the Hospital earned or received $2,577,377.73 and spent for operating expenses $2,494,191.24. This left $83,146.49 for the purchase of new equipment and alteration of two floors for civilian use.

Edgar Blake, Jr. Dies

The administration of Edgar Blake, Jr. at Wesley was relatively brief, five years and three days; yet his death from a heart condition on March 28, 1947, was a grievous shock. He was the son of a retired Methodist bishop and had been chief executive officer of the Methodist Hospital in Gary, Indiana, and a past president of the Indiana Hospital Association before joining Wesley as assistant superintendent November 1, 1941. He was appointed superintendent five months later. The leadership of Edgar Blake, Jr. through the tumultuous times of war-borne disorder and confusion to the well-organized, financially sound Wesley of 1947 merits special commendation in the Hospital's history.

Medical Staff Appointments

The remaining medical staff members had returned to their practices and teaching responsibilities, which had been increased by many young veterans seeking to resume postgraduate training. Dr. Gilbert H. Marquardt continued as chief of staff and announced the following appointments: Dr. Earl E. Barth, chairman, department of roentgenology; Dr. George H. Gardner, chairman, department of obstetrics and gynecology; Dr. William B. Wartman, chairman, department of pathology, and Dr. Thomas C. Laipply, pathologist.

New members appointed to the attending staff during 1946 were: Drs. George B. Bradburn, obstetrics and gynecology; Claire E. Carr, surgery; James A. Conner, pediatrics; Clinton L. Compere, orthopedics; David N. Danforth, obstetrics and gynecology; Edith Eason, anesthesia and oxygen therapy; Ronald R. Greene, obstetrics and gynecology; Arthur L. Juers, otolaryngology; Bertha A. Klein, ophthalmology; Walter G. Maddock, surgery; Elsie I. Wieczorowski, pediatrics, and Henry E. Wilson, Jr., medicine.

Dr. Marquardt reported that, since moving to the new building, Wesley's house staff has been increased from 16 to 64, 32 residents and 32 interns. The growth intensified a long-felt need for additional house staff living quarters and prompted the Board of Trustees to purchase the four-story building next door at 230 East Superior Street. The $80,000 structure provided convenient and attractive living quarters for interns and residents.

Hueston Heads Administration

Ralph M. Hueston, a veteran of 24 years in hospital administration, was appointed superintendent of Wesley effective July 14, 1947. He began in 1924 as superintendent of Cottage Hospital in Galesburg, Illinois for two years, followed by an administrative assignment at Austin Hospital (now Loretto Hospital) in Chicago before accepting the directorship of Silver Cross Hospital at Joliet, Illinois where he stayed nine years. In 1935 he became superintendent of Hurley Hospital in Flint, Michigan, and was an organizer and a trustee of the Blue Cross Plan for Michigan.

In announcing the new superintendent's appointment, the monthly publication, *Wesley MEMO*, disclosed that prior to his hospital affiliation, Hueston had been a vendor of hospital equipment in his native state, Iowa. In the course of business he met and married Beatrice L. Case, superintendent of the Eleanor Moore County Hospital in Boone, Iowa. The marriage, according to the story, was the beginning of Mr. Hueston's hospital career.

After the Hueston appointment, a young man with a promising future in hospital administration, Kenath Hartman, joined Wesley in February as administrative assistant. A month later he was married to Lorene Chow of the nursing faculty at Mt. Sinai Hospital and shortly thereafter he was promoted to assistant to the superintendent.

Hench Named President

Jay L. Hench, president of the Mid-West Forging and Manufacturing Co., and Wesley trustee since 1941, was elected president of the Hospital in early 1948, succeeding John Holmes who had served for six years. Hench worked first as an office boy, then salesman for Joseph T. Ryerson & Son before joining Lackawanna Steel Company in 1911 as assistant to the Chicago district manager, whom he succeeded. In 1922 Hench became associated with George Herbert Jones, donor of the Wesley building, to assist in management of companies controlled by Jones. As vice president, Hench developed the Mid-West Forging & Mfg. Co. Following the death of Mr. Jones in 1941, Mr. Hench became president and owner of the business.

Wesley Celebrates its 60th Anniversary

Six hundred men and women jammed the grand ballroom of the Lake Shore

Club on October 26, 1948, to pay homage to the sixtieth anniversary of Wesley's origin. The event attracted health and civic leaders, Wesley trustees, medical staff members, department heads and special guests.

The occasion recalled October 26, 1888, when a petition was filed with the Secretary of State of Illinois for approval to maintain Wesley Hospital in the City of Chicago, Illinois, "for the purpose of gratuitous treatment of diseases of the sick poor."

Bishop J. Ralph Magee opened the 1948 program with the invocation and Toastmaster Henry F. Tenney, a Wesley trustee, introduced guests at the speakers' table. Chicago Mayor Martin H. Kennelly paid tribute to Wesley's contributions to Chicago, saying "good hospitals, like good government, are a matter of importance and concern to the entire community." Dr. J. Roscoe Miller, president-elect of Northwestern University, spoke of Wesley's role in medical education. Chief of Staff Vincent J. O'Conor recalled achievements of Wesley physicians, naming several who had made medical history. President Jay L. Hench summarized important events in the Hospital since 1941 and explained that rising costs of providing care necessitated seeking outside financial aid for free bed care.

The program featured a pictorial pageant depicting Wesley's history and highlighting some of its current problems, narrated by Melvin Galliart, Chicago actor. Among the honored guests were Dr. William C. Danforth, son of Wesley's founder; Dr. Herman N. Bundesen, president of the Board of Health, City of Chicago; Joseph G. Norby, president of the American Hospital Association; Dean Conley, executive director of the American College of Hospital Administrators, and Dr. Malcolm T. MacEachern, associate director of the American College of Surgeons.

OTHER ANNIVERSARIES

The year 1948 contained two other significant anniversaries for one of Wesley's board members. It was the 40th year of Edwin L. Wagner's trusteeship, and the year that Mr. Wagner turned 80. A native of Polo, Illinois, Edwin Wagner came to Chicago at the age of 18 and was employed as a clerk in the old Metropolitan National Bank. He rose steadily in the banking profession and was a central figure in a number of bank mergers and reorganizations. He claimed that the most important merger of his career occurred in 1893, the year of the Columbian Exposition, when he married May Leslie, a Chicago girl.

After his retirement in 1932, Mr. Wagner devoted the major portion of his time to helping Wesley cope with its vexations. From 1937 to 1940 he donated his full time efforts to the problems of financing and planning a new building. In those days, Wesley, still recovering from the depression, had to pay its bills in installments. Mr. Wagner personally persuaded many a supplier to allow the Hospital a little more time to meet its obligations. Only a few months after the anniversary dinner, Wesley's trustee of longest tenure, Edwin L. Wagner, died February 16, 1949.

Dixon Grill Opens

Another festive occasion during the 60th anniversary year was the opening of the Dixon Grill, named for the family who had served Wesley for three generations. For the past half century there had been at least one Dixon trustee, more often three, their aggregate trusteeships totaling 117 years by 1948. During that year the Dixon board members were George W. Dixon, vice-president; Homer L. Dixon, and George W. Dixon, Jr. In 1949 Wesley M. Dixon, president of the Container Corporation of America, was elected to fill the vacancy left by the death of Edwin L. Wagner. In addition, Dixon wives and daughters served in many capacities with the women's groups and on the Board of Trustees.

The attractive mirror-paneled Dixon Grill with green and black motif on white at once became a popular luncheon and snack rendezvous for personnel, volunteers and visitors.

Chaplain Appointed; Chapel Dedicated

In 1948, a man was appointed who would serve Wesley as its chaplain for more than a quarter of a century—the Reverend Robert A. Dahl. Born and reared in Oak Park, Illinois, Dahl had been minister of the Union Park Methodist Church in Des Moines, Iowa. In ministering to spiritual needs at Wesley, the Reverend Dahl visited an average of 40 patients a day and notified pastors of church members in the Hospital.

On Easter Sunday, 1949, the Reverend Dahl officiated at the dedication of Wesley's new chapel on the ninth floor. Here Sunday services for patients were conducted as well as devotional programs for student nurses, small weddings and memorial services. A beautiful stained glass window with a Biblical scene, gift of the Nurse Alumnae Association, ornamented the chapel which was built entirely by hospital carpenters.

WESLEY HONORS NUMS DEAN

Dr. Richard H. Young, new dean of Northwestern University Medical School, was Wesley's honored guest at a dinner in the Hospital's Peacock Room on August 11, 1949, to officially welcome him to the university's Chicago campus. Other guests were Dr. J. Roscoe Miller, new president of Northwestern University; Richard Vanderwarker, director of Passavant Memorial Hospital; Ralph M. Hueston, superintendent of Wesley, and the medical staff executive committee members of both Passavant and Wesley hospitals.

Dr. Young succeeded Dr. Miller, who had been medical school dean since 1941. Dr. Miller was elected to the Wesley Board of Trustees, filling the vacancy left by Dr. Snyder when he retired. Before coming to Northwestern, Dr. Young was dean of the College of Medicine of the University of Utah.

NURSING SCHOOL AND DEPARTMENTS EXPAND

Terminating the United States Cadet Nurse Corps at the end of the war did not cause a drop in applicants to the Wesley School of Nursing as anticipated. WAVEs, WACs and SPARs applied for admission to the school as well as to the Hospital's course for medical record librarians. The majority of student nurse anesthetists were former army and navy nurses.

By 1949 Wesley's nursing school had grown to 300 students and nursing personnel numbered 235. Edna S. Newman was named director of both the Wesley School of Nursing and Nursing Service replacing Harriet H. Smith, who had resigned after five years.

Miss Newman had been director of the school of nursing and nursing service at Cook County Hospital for 11 years. She also had been assistant professor of nursing education at the University of Chicago and assistant director of nurses at the Illinois Training School for Nurses.

A nurse aide course was introduced by the nursing department and directed by Edith Chambers to train aides to perform routine bedside duties to free registered nurses to care for the critically ill and perform other professional nursing services.

Wesley's business office had grown in proportion to its service and required a key executive to manage business and financial operations. Donald A. Bloom, a certified public accountant, was appointed comptroller in 1948 to head a department of 129 persons including admitting, payroll, accounting, credit, and telephone services. Bloom had specialized in accounting at Antioch College in Yellow Springs, Ohio, where students trained at companies during part of the school year. He was assigned to an accounting firm where he continued working after graduation and became a CPA. During the war Bloom was a headquarters supply officer with the rank of captain, at Randolph Field, Texas, and in Hawaii.

In Memoriam

Wesley lost a valuable and devoted medical staff member and employee in the untimely death of Dr. Helen M. Patton August 4, 1948. Helen Patton came to Wesley as a student nurse in 1923, was graduated three years later and became supervisor of the men's ward. In 1928 she went to Wichita, Kansas to work as a surgical supervisor. Her desire for further medical knowledge brought her back to Chicago where she became a student and medical research assistant at Northwestern. She was graduated with Phi Beta Kappa honors and a B.S. degree in 1936.

Miss Patton continued her research at the medical school for several years before enrolling as a medical student. She received her M.D. degree in 1943 and returned to Wesley for her internship, then her residency. She was appointed instructor of medicine at Northwestern, member of the attending staff at Wesley and administrative assistant to the hospital superintendent. In the latter capacity she directed house staff activities, was administrative head of the health service, emergency, anesthesia and photography departments. Her contributions to medicine and to hospital administration as well as her gracious human qualities were remembered with affection by all who knew her.

Learning While Healing　　　Chapter 18

esley's second decade on Northwestern University's Chicago campus began with its educational programs an integral part of its total service, far surpassing its original commitment to the university. In addition to the normal daily traffic of patients, doctors, employees and visitors, some 500 students came to the Hospital with books in arms or in uniforms prepared for on-the-job training. There were medical graduates serving internships and residencies, young women soon to be registered nurses, and others studying to be nurse anesthetists, laboratory technicians, medical record librarians and hospital administrators.

Wesley considered the care of patients to be its primary function. Therefore the Hospital accepted a responsibility to assist in educating not only the physicians, as agreed in its affiliation with Northwestern, but others who served the patients.

A total of 189 Northwestern medical students participated in Wesley's 1952 medical education program. Second year medical students were assigned to the pathology department where groups of 25 met in the autopsy amphitheater for instruction and demonstration. All students, including freshmen, attended the weekly presentation of autopsy material, microscopic sections, and the biweekly clinical pathological conference. Junior medical students were assigned to case studies and lectures by hospital staff members who also were on Northwestern's faculty. Senior medical students became clinical clerks at Wesley where they recorded case histories and gained rapport with patients.

Each of Wesley's 32 interns spent a year on rotating assignments in obstetrics and various specialties of medicine and surgery, including anesthesiology, otolaryngology, gynecology, neurosurgery, orthopedics, neuropsychiatry and urology. Wesley offered residencies in each of the above specialties as well as in internal medicine, general surgery, ophthalmology, pathology and radiology. Each of Wesley's 45 residents served a year in his chosen specialty as active assistant to attending physicians and in supervising and instructing interns and medical students. Residents also were assigned periodically to the outpatient department of the Montgomery Ward Clinic at Northwestern Medical School.

THE SCHOOL OF NURSING

Wesley's affiliation with Northwestern gave the Hospital's 300 student nurses the option of taking the three-year course for the diploma of graduate nurse, or the combined liberal arts and nursing program leading to the bachelor of science degree and graduate nurse diploma.

During the preclinical period, the first six months of training, students learned basic nursing skills and studied general medical courses. Success brought acceptance as clinical students and they received their caps—symbol of the nursing profession. They worked in the medical and surgical wards, diet kitchen and central service department, and attended classes and lectures. The second and third years were spent in specialized areas such as surgery, obstetrics, psychiatry and pediatrics.

The school had two affiliations—with the Illinois Neuropsychiatric Institute where students gained psychiatric nursing experience, and with Children's Memorial Hospital where they were trained in pediatric nursing. The Wesley School of Nursing received funds for scholarships from the Woman's Auxiliary, the Service League, Wesley Nurses' Alumnae Association, Charles Ward Seaburg Fund, Chicago Council on Community Nursing and the Lizzie K. Schermerhorn Fund.

Two graduates of the Class of 1951 earned the highest grades in the examination for nurse registration given by the Illinois State Department of Registration and Education. Alice Gugeler, 23, of Burlington, Iowa, received the highest grade of all nurses taking the examination in Illinois;

Margy Dillon, 22, of Provo, Utah, made the second highest mark. Both young women received diplomas in nursing from Wesley's school in March and their bachelor of science degrees from Northwestern University's college of liberal arts in June. Both joined the nursing staff at Wesley.

The Wesley School of Nursing, one of the largest in the country, had a faculty of 60 graduate nurses of whom 21 taught full time, plus a registrar, librarian, housemother, counselor and director. The entire program was under the guidance of Edna S. Newman, who had been appointed director of nursing service and the school of nursing in October, 1948. Prior to joining Wesley, she had held the same position at the Cook County Hospital. A graduate of the Philadelphia General Hospital School of Nursing, she held an M.A. degree from Teachers College, Columbia University.

The National Nursing Accrediting Service notified Superintendent Hueston that the Wesley Memorial Hospital School of Nursing was granted accreditation for 1952. The NNAS was a joint association of the professional nursing organizations which approved programs of nursing education conducted by hospitals, colleges and universities. Application for accreditation was voluntary and approval indicated that the school met recognized standards. Only about ten percent of nursing schools in the country were accredited at that time.

SCHOOL FOR NURSE ANESTHETISTS

At least six student nurses were trained each year in the art of anesthesia under the direction of Dr. Mary L. Karp, senior attending physician and chairman of the department of anesthesia and oxygen therapy. Each of the staff of 14 anesthesiologists and nurse anesthetists, who served Wesley's approximately 10,000 surgery patients yearly, also was responsible for working with students individually and in groups.

Anesthesia had progressed rapidly since its discovery in 1846, becoming more complicated with each advance in surgery, the life-saving skill made possible by the pain-killing agents. Students learned the chemical formula of each agent—when, where, how and why it was used—and they assisted in administering general and local anesthesia. Surgery had not reached the complexity of open-heart, transplant and microsurgical operations, but its companion specialty—anesthesia—was setting the stage.

Nurse anesthetists were trained to use the iron lung for polio patients in the days before the Salk vaccine when the dreaded disease was crippling hundreds of Chicago children. They also were schooled in inhalation therapy before that method of treatment became an individual department in most hospitals.

SCHOOL OF MEDICAL TECHNOLOGY

Medical advances of the past 25 years had multiplied the need for medical technicians, 36 of whom were employed by Wesley alone. In 1952, Wesley's School of Medical Technology, a term relatively unknown in 1925, was among 400 throughout the country offering medical technical training. At Wesley, the classrooms were the five laboratories where skill was acquired through on-the-job training. Students learned to make blood counts, prepare tissue for miscroscopic slides, prepare blood plasma, give basal metabolism tests and take electrocardiograms. Students attended special lecture courses in chemistry, hematology and bacteriology.

Eighteen students were enrolled in the school and received certificates after completion. All were successful in the final hurdle, the registration examination given by the American Society of Clinical Pathologists.

SCHOOL FOR MEDICAL RECORDS LIBRARIANS

The medical records librarian had a demanding obligation to the patient, his physician and the hospital. The patient's case history—a summary of his care—was of vital importance to him, particularly if he returned to the hospital, and to his physician and others who cared for him. Medical records were essential in case of a law suit, indispensable to medical research and to the hospital itself. The efficiency of the medical records department was an influential factor in a hospital's accreditation by the Joint Commission on Accreditation of Hospitals. These facts dictated the curriculum planned by Marjorie Quandt, instructor and department director, for the students who came each year from various parts of the country to take the one-year course.

Records librarian students learned medical terminology, library science and basic legal aspects of hospital service. They took courses in anatomy and physiology, studied various types of diseases and injuries, and became familiar with diagnostic methods.

Upon successful completion of the course at Wesley, students earned a certificate in medical library science qualifying them to take the national registry examination. Those who passed became an R.R.L., Registered Records Librarian, qualified for work in hospitals, clinics, public health departments and industrial plants.

Something new was added to Wesley's medical records department in December, 1951, when the Hospital became the first in Chicago to install the Edison "Televoicewriter." The machine enabled a surgeon to dictate the record of an operation immediately after completion through a special telephone at any of four locations. The phones were on special lines direct to the medical records library where typists transposed records to written form and had them properly filed.

RESIDENCY PROGRAM IN HOSPITAL ADMINISTRATION

The profession of hospital administration was a fairly recent development and Wesley had been one of the first hospitals offering residencies to students who had received formal training in the field at a medical school.

In 1943 when Dr. Malcolm T. MacEachern, one of the founders of the movement for acccreditation of hospitals, established a hospital administration course at Northwestern University Medical School there was only one other such program in the country: at the University of Chicago. In 1945 a hospital administration course was started at Columbia University in New York followed in rapid succession by the University of Minnesota, Washington University at St. Louis, Johns Hopkins and Yale Universities.[1]

The American Hospital Association and the American College of Hospital Administrators encouraged the programs and suggested curriculum content to provide opportunities for hundreds of young men and women who had gained some hospital administrative experience in the armed forces and were interested in the field as a career.

At Wesley the residency program was tailored to meet the candidate's specific needs. Under the guidance of Superintendent Ralph M Hueston, the resident learned the operation of a hospital as a whole and the functions and problems of individual departments. He observed the teamwork and cooperation among the doctors, nurses and employees as they combined their skills to care for patients. He learned that education and research

[1] *Ray E. Brown, Graduate Education for Hospital Administration*

complement patient care and he became aware of the grave responsibility accepted by the administrative staff.

After meeting the academic requirements of the school's classroom program and the hospital's on-the-job training, the student earned a master's degree in Hospital Administration.

Board of Trustees Enlarged

Early in 1951 the Wesley Board of Trustees had voted to change the bylaws to provide for an increase in the number of trustees from 30 to 36. New trustees were elected including Paul C. Clovis, president and director, 20th Century Press, Inc.; Arthur Dole, Jr., president and director, Hooker Glass and Paint Mfg. Co.; Wrigley Offield, William Wrigley, Jr. Company; Harold A. Smith, Winston Strawn, Shaw & Black, attorneys, and Samuel W. Witwer, Jr., Wilkinson, Witwer & Moran, attorneys. Henry Loeppert, president of Boyd-Wagner Company, became a trustee the following year.

Shortly before the change in bylaws, the Board of Trustees had lost a loyal and devoted member of 27 years, Homer Laing Dixon, 69, son of Arthur Dixon, the original Dixon trustee. At the time of Homer's death, October 1, 1950, two of his nephews, George W. and Wesley M., were Wesley trustees.

Old Wesley Sold; New Wesley Debt Free

The sale of Old Wesley, an action under negotiation for two years, was closed February 7, 1952, when the City of Chicago agreed to pay $32,250 for the old Wesley Hospital and adjoining property. The building was razed to make way for a Chicago housing project.

Proceeds from the sale were used to help retire the mortgage that had been placed on the hospital properties to finance the completion and equip the new Wesley. The final payment was made on the house staff residence on May 14, 1952, leaving Wesley free of all mortgage debts.

At the annual meeting of the Board of Trustees January 10, 1953, James F. Stiles, Jr., chairman and treasurer of Abbott Laboratories, was elected president, succeeding Jay L. Hench who had served for five years. On the following May 8, Mr. Stiles was cited as "Industrial Man of the Year" at the annual convention of the National Council of Industrial Management Clubs at Grand Rapids, Michigan.

WESLEY ALUMNI JOIN STAFF

Dr. Samuel J. Fogelson, surgeon, who had been elected chief of staff in 1950, emphasized the many Wesley-trained doctors who had joined the staff. They included Carl E. Billings, Charles I. Fisher, Frederic A. Lestina and Jacques M. Smith, medicine; Melvyn A. Bayly and Ben M. Peckham, obstetrics and gynecology; Erich Liebert, neuropsychiatry; Orville E. Gordon and Frank W. Newell, ophthalmology.

Another staff member who had served his residency at Wesley, Dr. Abram H. Cannon, was appointed chairman of the department of radiology after Dr. Earl E. Barth resigned to enter the private practice of roentgenology. Before receiving his M.D. degree from Northwestern, Dr. Cannon had attended the University of Utah, later returning to Salt Lake City to intern at Latter Day Saints Hospital.

Dr. Thomas C. Laipply, chairman of Wesley's pathology department, was named director of the medical services department in July 1950. The position originated with Dr. Helen Patton who had been responsible for the administration of professional services including the medical education program until her sudden death in 1948. Dr. Henry Wilson, director of Northwestern's Montgomery Ward Clinics, assumed the department's responsibilities with the assistance of Dr. James B. O'Neill for an interim period. As medical services director, Dr. Laipply accepted full responsibility for planning and supervising Wesley's entire medical education program for medical clerks, interns, residents and fellows.

Three young doctors who were strangers when they arrived as interns at Wesley July 1, 1950, had a common bond as candidates selected by the Methodist Church for its Crusade Scholars program for the foreign mission field. Dr. Friedrich C. Tross of Innsbruck, Austria, Dr. Stepheno Ammenti of Zurich, Switzerland, and Dr. Wolfgang F. Kollert of Nuremberg, Germany, had the distinction of being the only medical doctors among 150 promising students selected. Upon completion of the year's internship, all three planned to enter missionary work in Africa, the Belgian Congo, Angola or Liberia.

DOUBLE CHAIRMANSHIPS

Dr. Benjamin Boshes, professor and chairman of the department of nervous and mental diseases at Northwestern, was appointed chairman of Wesley's department of neuropsychiatry in October, 1953. He succeeded Dr. Theodore T. Stone who died March 5, 1952.

Dr. Norman G. Parry, Wesley chief of staff for 1953, commented that the appointment of Dr. Boshes brought to five the number of doctors who were chairmen of the same departments at both Wesley and Northwestern. The others were Dr. Edward L. Compere, chairman of the Wesley department of orthopedics and of the Northwestern department of bone and joint surgery; Dr. George H. Gardner, chairman of the departments of obstetrics and gynecology; Dr. George E. Shambaugh, Jr., chairman of the departments of otolaryngology; and Dr. Vincent J. O'Conor, chairman of the departments of urology.

CHICAGO WESLEY MEMORIAL HOSPITAL IS FORMED

Negotiations to merge Wesley Memorial Hospital and Chicago Memorial Hospital began in the spring of 1953 and ended June 30, 1954 when the combined institution, Chicago Wesley Memorial Hospital, was announced.

The boards of trustees of the two hospitals were united, forming a board with 39 trustees. Eleven physicians of the Chicago Memorial Hospital were appointed to the Wesley medical staff. Added to Wesley's assets of $8,889,431, as published in the treasurer's report for 1954, were Chicago Memorial's assets: endowment funds approximating $2,098,000; free care funds approximating $400,000 and properties at 660 East Groveland estimated to sell for $500,000. Equal ranks of the Chicago Memorial physicians were transferred from the University of Illinois, where they were affiliated, to Northwestern University.

As many of Chicago Memorial personnel as could be assimilated in the combined hospital were employed in comparable positions within the established salary range at Wesley.

Dr. H. Ivan Sippy, Wesley chief of staff for 1954-1955 and himself a transferred physician from Washington Boulevard Hospital, graciously welcomed the newcomers in his annual report for the medical staff:

> "Future historians of Wesley will not pass lightly over the year 1954, during which eventful developments have had a remarkable concentration.

"The Medical Staff and Courtesy Group have been strengthened by our most welcome new members from the Chicago Memorial Hospital. These are: Dr. Sam W. Banks, orthopedics; Dr. Paul C. Bucy, surgery (chief of neurosurgical section); Dr. Michael C. Govostis, surgery; Dr. Richard E. Heller, surgery; Dr. Jerome D. Kaufman, obstetrics and gynecology; Dr. H. R. Oberhill, surgery; Dr. Gordon Scott, otolaryngology; Dr. T. A. Wozniak, orthopedics; Dr. Fred Miller, Courtesy Group, surgery; and Dr. Walter N. Wiborg, Courtesy Group, surgery.

"This new affiliation is already proving as pleasant and advantageous to all concerned as did the similar merging with the staff of Washington Boulevard Hospital in 1942.

"Other new members acquired in 1954, by promotion or appointment, and also cordially welcomed are, for the staff: Dr. Edward Avery, surgery; Dr. Arthur DeBoer, surgery; Dr. Wiley Harrison, otolaryngology; Dr. Theodore Hudson, surgery; Dr. Paul Kezdi, medicine; Dr. Raymond Langenbach, medicine; Dr. Francis J. Tenczar, pathology; Dr. John L. Reichert, pediatrics; and for the Courtesy Group: Dr. Robert G. Addison, orthopedics; Dr. Leon A. Carrow, obstetrics and gynecology; Dr. William B. Fischer, orthopedics; Dr. Constance Graves, anesthesiology; Dr. Walter E. Hagens, ophthalmology; Dr. Warren W. Kreft, ophthalmology; Dr. Verner E. Lamb, anesthesiology; Dr. Orion H. Stuteville, otolaryngology; Dr. Arthur Sweet, orthopedics; and Dr. Robert G. Thompson, orthopedics."

Chicago Memorial Hospital had another asset—an interesting history. The hospital had been established for the Hahnemann Medical College of Chicago for which the charter had been drawn up in the law offices of Abraham Lincoln in Springfield in 1850. The college taught the principles of homeopathy, a theory which stressed therapeutics or cures rather than etiology or causes of disease.[1] The theory was originated in Germany by Samuel Hahnemann and brought to Philadelphia where the Hahnemann Medical School and Hospital was established in 1843. Homeopathy spread and gained followers, especially in Chicago where some 500 homeopaths practiced in 1900. However, the doctrines of Robert Koch, Louis Pasteur and Joseph Lister had become known and understood. The pathogenic role of bacteria was irrefutable and methods of asepsis and antisepsis were universally accepted. The old beliefs and techniques died out and the Hahnemann Medical College of Chicago was closed in 1922.

[1] *William H. King, ed. History of Homeopathy and its Institutions in America, Chicago, 1905*

The hospital, which had been founded by such influential Chicagoans as J. Young Scammon, John Wentworth, and William B. Ogden, continued to serve its community. The name was changed to Chicago Memorial Hospital and its medical staff adopted regular medical techniques. Later the hospital became associated with the University of Illinois.

After the merger June 30, 1954, a bronze plaque 24 inches wide and 48 inches long was placed in the lobby of Chicago Wesley Memorial Hospital with the following inscription:

In Commemoration of

The Hahnemann Hospital of the City of Chicago
organized February 14, 1855
and of
Chicago Memorial Hospital
Successor, by change of name January 24, 1924
Merged June 30, 1954 with

Wesley Memorial Hospital into

Chicago Wesley Memorial Hospital

Resolution

Whereas the Hahnemann Hospital of the City of Chicago was organized February 14, 1855 by special charter adopted by the Illinois General Assembly and prepared and sponsored with the aid of Abraham Lincoln.

And whereas said Hospital operated continuously until January 24, 1924 when the name was changed to Chicago Memorial Hospital and thereafter until June 30, 1954 when it merged with Wesley Memorial Hospital into Chicago Wesley Memorial Hospital.

Be it further resolved that recognition be and it is hereby given all who, according to the preserved records of said Hospital, were devoted to said Hospital and community as evidenced by personal services and by contributions of funds and property, and particularly by:

Dr. George E. Shipman who founded said Hospital; Mrs. William H. Wright, Mrs. Caroline E. Haskell, J. Young Scammon, Mayor of Chicago; Robert Allerton, William L. Brown, Dr. Robert R. Chislete, George E. P.

Dodge, Dr. R. Reuben Ludlam, George E. McCammon, Erskine E. Phelps, Dr. Steven Seymour, James P. Soper, Edward F. Swift, Catherine M. White, William Wrigley, Jr., David B. and Louis M. Shipman, and many others who endowed the Hospital.

Raymond M. Ashcraft, Vernon R. Loucks, Henry J. McFarland, John J. Mitchell, John E. Wilder who, as presidents of the Board gave generously of their time, talents and money.

Dr. George E. Shears, member of the medical staff, board and superintendent and responsible for substantial gifts.

Josephine Blalock, Mrs. Valentine R. Bosworth, superintendents, Cora Oberholt, superintendent of nurses training school.

New Needs Arise at Wesley

One of the advantages of the merger was the combined endowment and trust funds of the two hospitals. The increased income made possible larger allocations for care of indigent patients. Before the merger, Wesley's monthly expense for free care was $8,000, a sum which was raised to $11,000 a month immediately after the merger. The sale of the Chicago Memorial Hospital building and property to the Chicago Land Clearance Commission for $250,000 was consummated August 15, 1955.

Prior to the merger, Wesley had acquired property at 224-220 East Superior Street from the American Dental Association at a cost of $325,000. In 1955 the purchase of property at 228 East Superior Street completed the acquisition of land between the Hospital and the ADA building. This gave Wesley a building site of 80 feet frontage on East Superior Street with a depth of 125 feet.

These actions of the Board of Trustees proved timely. During the 14 years that Wesley had occupied its cathedral-type building, numerous services with appropriate equipment had been added. These were essential to stay abreast of the rapid medical advances during and following World War II. The need for space was restricting patient care in almost every department, an intolerable situation. To meet the obvious need, the trustees in 1954 engaged the architects, Fugard, Burt, Wilkinson and Orth to prepare expansion plans. The firm succeeded Thielbar and Fugard, architects of the Cathedral of Healing.

Building for Better Service   Chapter 19

Wesley's need for expansion in all areas of hospital service in 1954 was evaluated by the Board of Trustees, who lost no time in initiating a development program. The three-point plan included constructing a new addition, purchasing a building for living quarters of married house staff members and remodeling the existing building. Cost of the entire program was estimated at $7,500,000. Wesley had on hand about $2,500,000 available for expansion and a federal grant of $200,000 to aid in building. About $4,800,000 was needed and the trustees decided that for the first time in its 67 years of service, the Hospital would invite the public to participate in a fund raising campaign. Former Wesley President John Holmes, chairman of the board and chief executive officer of Swift & Company, was named campaign chairman. Committee members were James F. Stiles, Jr., president of Wesley and chairman of the board of Abbott Laboratories; Vernon R. Loucks, attorney, and William H. Mitchell, senior partner in Mitchell, Hutchins and Company, investment firm, all Wesley trustees. Those leading the division for memorial gifts were Harold A. Smith, Samuel W. Witwer, Henry V. Loeppert and Bishop J. Ralph Magee. Heading the medical division were Drs. H. Ivan Sippy, Arthur E. Mahle, Samuel J. Fogelson and Richard A. Perritt.

The campaign was launched September 28, 1955, when Wesley friends gathered at the Lake Shore Club for the kickoff dinner. After a brief outline of the development program, particularly its major feature, the new addition, Dr. Gilbert H. Marquardt made a joyful announcement: "A gift of one million dollars has been given toward the new addition. However, I am not at liberty to give the name of the generous donor at this time."

It was revealed later that the benefactor was Mrs. William M. (Ruth Jones) Allison, whom propriety had prompted to request anonymity while she was present—and she did want to attend the dinner. Mrs. Allison, a member of the Wesley Board of Trustees, was continuing the work of her father, George Herbert Jones, whose gift of $3,500,000 had made possible the Cathedral of Healing in 1941.

Ground breaking was held May 11, 1956, a dark and cloudy day, when Wesley associates and friends gathered on the northeast side of the existing building for the ceremony. Mrs. Allison turned the first spadeful of earth assisted by Wesley President Stiles. The rain held off until Bishop Charles W. Brashares pronounced the benediction, then a downpour sent everyone scurrying for shelter.

While excavation was under way, the trustees accomplished another part of the development program. They concluded on June 4, 1956, the purchase of a seven-story, L-shaped building at 222 East Delaware Place to provide urgently needed apartments for married interns and residents. The building, located just four blocks from Wesley, contained 38 apartments of appropriate size for moderate-priced housing.

THE RUTH JONES ALLISON PAVILION
The general contractor for the addition, Gust K. Newberg Construction Company, made rapid progress and started the superstructure in mid-October, 1956, eight weeks ahead of schedule. As the concrete and steel work rose and plans for the cornerstone laying were made, one of Wesley's most beloved patrons, Mrs. Allison, became ill and was confined to her bed. Her interest and generosity had served as inspiration to many, and everyone associated with Wesley was bereaved when her death occurred on February 1, 1957. Not only had she led the way for the new addition with a million dollar gift, but she also had established the patient library in the main building and had served countless hours as a dedicated volunteer. The

Board of Trustees paid tribute to this gracious lady by naming the new addition the Ruth Jones Allison Pavilion.

In the February, 1957, issue of *Wesley MEMO*, the Hospital's employee publication, John R. Kinsey, public relations director and editor, wrote the following editorial under the heading, In Memory of Mrs. Allison:

"Ruth Jones Allison was a wonderful woman. She was the kind of a woman who on one day would be consulted by leading Chicagoans about important plans for the opera season—and the next day could be seen talking with our doorman and being more concerned about his health than about opera stars...We all know of her extreme generosity to Wesley—the magnificent gift to our building fund, establishing the Patients' Library, providing books and magazines, furnishing the Stork Club for expectant fathers, contributing furniture and a steady supply of flowers and plants, to mention some of her deeds...

"But not too many people know about the "little" things that she did almost every day to bring happiness to others. One day she learned that a former Wesley employee had a fine voice and that an operatic career seemed possible if the girl could receive proper training. Mrs. Allison helped make it possible for her to study and today this young woman is a successful vocalist. We are referring to Marilyn Powell who sang at the memorial services and afterward told the *MEMO* editor, 'I would be glad for you to put in the article that Mrs. Allison helped me.'

"...And she had a sense of humor. After her million dollar gift to our building fund was announced, she consented to an interview. One reporter asked, 'Mrs. Allison, would you consider me impertinent if I asked your age?'

"She smiled slightly. Her eyes twinkled. Then she said, 'Yes.' All the reporters, and Mrs. Allison, chuckled—and the subject was dropped. As we said at the beginning, Mrs. Allison was a wonderful woman."

ARTHUR DOLE ELECTED PRESIDENT

As construction progressed on the Allison Pavilion, administrative and medical procedures continued within the Hospital. Arthur Dole, Jr., president of Hooker Glass and Paint Manufacturing Company, was elected president of the Wesley Board of Trustees at its annual meeting January 11, 1958. He succeeded James F. Stiles, Jr., president for five years, who had accepted the position of National Director of the United States Treasury's Savings Bond Division. In that capacity he became Assistant Secretary of the Treasury.

HEART SURGERY NATIONALLY ACCLAIMED
Dr. Arthur E. Mahle, internist, who was elected chief of the medical staff
in 1956, stated in the following year's annual report:

> "Under the guidance of Dr. Paul Kezdi and members of the Heart Station
> and Electrocardiology Department, Wesley has made striking advances in
> diagnostic procedures related to diseases of the heart and blood vessels.
>
> "This department, aside from the recording of electrocardiograms and
> their interpretation, includes such activities as the diagnostic evaluation of
> patients by means of clinical and cardiac catherization findings...The staff
> members assist during surgery of the heart in operations which only a few
> years ago were unknown but during the last few years have restored to
> normal activity many 'hopeless' cardiac patients.
>
> "The acquisition of a new x-ray machine allows the examiner to do the
> delicate operation of catherization without darkening the room. It further
> aids in taking rapid moving pictures during the test for better evalua-
> tion...The heart station has received funds from the Schermerhorn Memo-
> rial Fund, the United States Public Health Service and the Life Insurance
> Research Fund. This department is looking forward with great expectations
> to the move into the new wing of the hospital where the heart station will
> have ample space to carry out increased activities."

Wesley had been nationally known for heart work for some time. In
February, 1954, Chicago newspapers published articles about a new type of
heart operation performed at Wesley described as "one of the most difficult
surgical procedures ever created."

The first of its type ever performed in Chicago, the two-stage operation
was developed to alleviate coronary artery disease, said to be the most
common of all heart ailments and the No. 1 cause of death in the United
States at that time. The patient was a 59-year-old Chicago factory worker
who formerly was a college professor and member of parliament in pre-war
Yugoslavia, who had fled communism.

Four months earlier Chicago newspapers and national wire services
carried stories on a new type of heart operation which Wesley surgeons used
to aid patients with auricular septal defects (abnormal opening between the
two upper chambers of the heart).

METABOLIC RESEARCH ADVANCED

Metabolic research was accelerated at Wesley in 1956 through a $147,000 grant from the John A. Hartford Foundation, established by John A. Hartford, for many years president of the Atlantic & Pacific Tea Company. The first research projects conducted under grant were:

(1) A study of nitrogen metabolism and amino acid requirements of patients with severely impaired renal function.

(2) The effect of salicylates on the plasma and urinary steroids of healthy subjects and patients with rheumatoid arthritis.

These and other projects were carried on during 1956 through 1958, the period covered by the grant. The research staff included Dr. Smith Freeman, chairman of the biochemistry department of Northwestern University; Dr. Richard Herndon, a resident physician at Wesley; and Dr. Anne S. Cleveland, of the University of California, whose services were shared by Wesley and Northwestern.

ALLISON PAVILION: HOSPITAL OF THE FUTURE

Five years of planning and building plus outstanding public support brought the Ruth Jones Allison Pavilion to completion. Dedication ceremonies were held March 16, 1959, two years and ten months after the ground breaking. Wesley President Arthur Dole, Jr., presided at the program in the solarium with the following participants:

Dr. J. Roscoe Miller, president, Northwestern University; John Duba, assistant mayor of Chicago; Dr. Joseph F. Mallach, chief of staff; Dr. Richard H. Young, dean, Northwestern University Medical School; Dr. Herman N. Bundesen, president, Board of Health; Dorsey R. Crowe, alderman, 42nd Ward; Ralph M. Hueston, hospital superintendent; the Reverend Charles Wesley Brashares, bishop, Methodist Church; and the Reverend Robert A. Dahl, chaplain. William M. Allison, husband of the structure's late donor, cut the traditional ribbon at the Chicago Avenue entrance to the new pavilion.

Following the ceremony, hundreds of guests toured the beautiful new building which already was in use. The five-story L-shaped building, facing Chicago Avenue and bordering Fairbanks Court, was used exclusively for hospital services and the 15-story tower contained both patients' rooms and doctors' offices. It was the first time in Chicago that doctors' offices were installed within a hospital. The overall floor space was increased by 55 percent and beds for patients from 617 to approximately 700. Both the pathology laboratories and the diagnostic x-ray laboratories were doubled in size and contained a vast array of new equipment. X-ray therapy contained the latest and largest units, including the $60,000 Curie cobalt unit for treatment of deep-seated tumors.

Guests toured the new psychiatric unit for 49 patients, recovery room for 18 patients, physical medicine department, heart station, pharmacy, and 6,000 square feet of research laboratories. They visited the new chapel, the administrative offices, the new patients' library, the classrooms and even the tunnel connecting the Allison Pavilion with the Medical School. These splendid new facilities enabled Wesley physicians to apply the latest known medical techniques in diagnosis and treatment, greatly improving service to a larger number of patients. The press hailed the $6.5 million Ruth Jones Allison Pavilion as the unit which set the pattern for future hospitals.

PERSONNEL APPOINTMENTS
Several changes in key personnel took place before and after the building program began. The nursing department had been under new leadership since September, 1954, when E. Elizabeth Geiger succeeded Edna S. Newman, who retired after five years as director of nursing.

Miss Geiger was a graduate of Wesley's school of nursing and held a bachelor of science and a master's degree in nursing from Teachers College, Columbia University, New York. She joined the administrative staff of the school of nursing at Cook County Hospital in 1947 and became director of its nursing service and school of nursing in 1949.

Agnes M. Spangler, a teacher from LaGrange, worked in the gift shop for two years before becoming director of volunteers in 1957. She succeeded Elizabeth Lundy, who resigned after four years to become director of the health museum at the Hinsdale Medical Center.

RESIDENTS IN HOSPITAL ADMINISTRATION
Wesley's administrative offices served as training grounds for students of Northwestern's hospital administration course. A succession of young men assisted in administration while gaining experience for hospital careers.

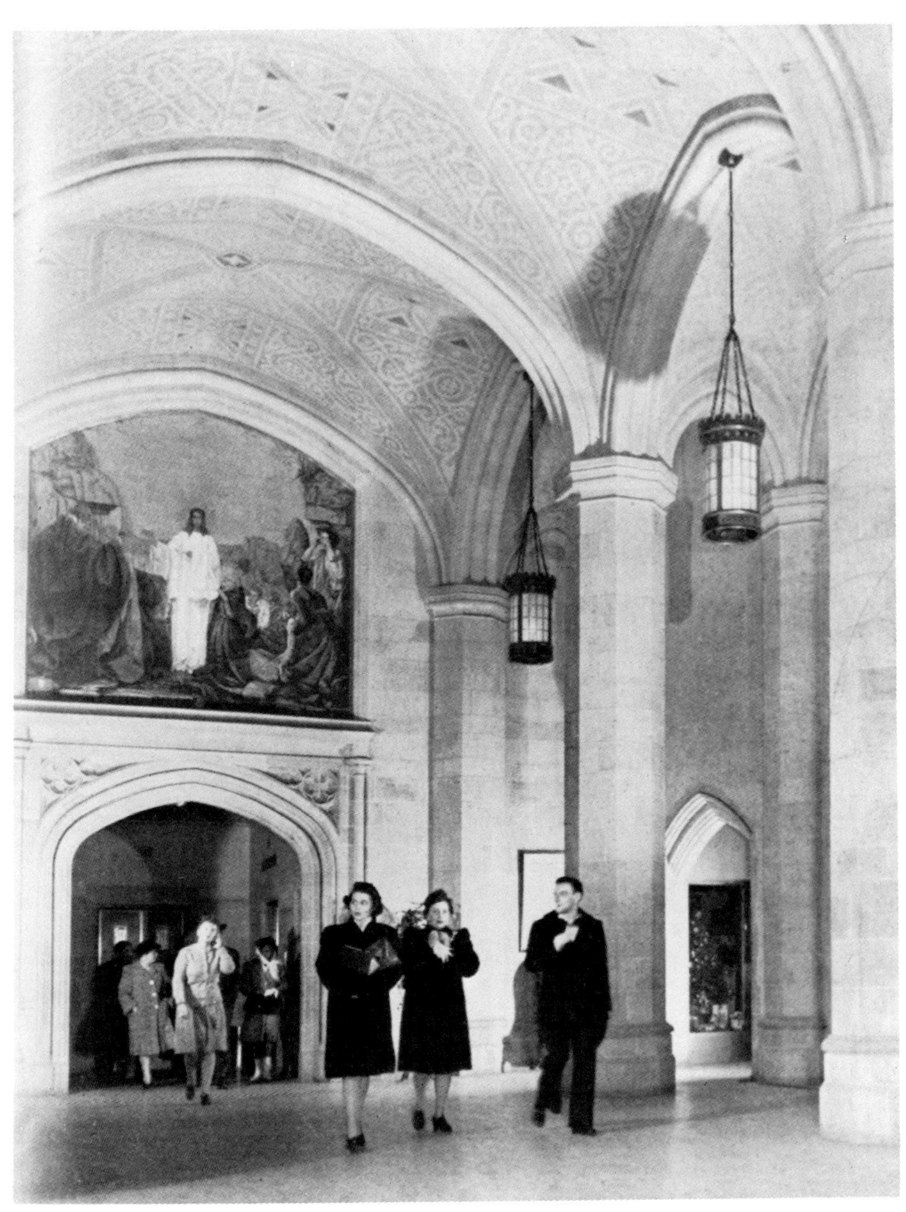

*Wesley's Cathedral of Healing with marble
floors and vaulted ceilings, was dedicated
November 30, 1941, beneath the gold leaf
mural,* The Divine Healer.

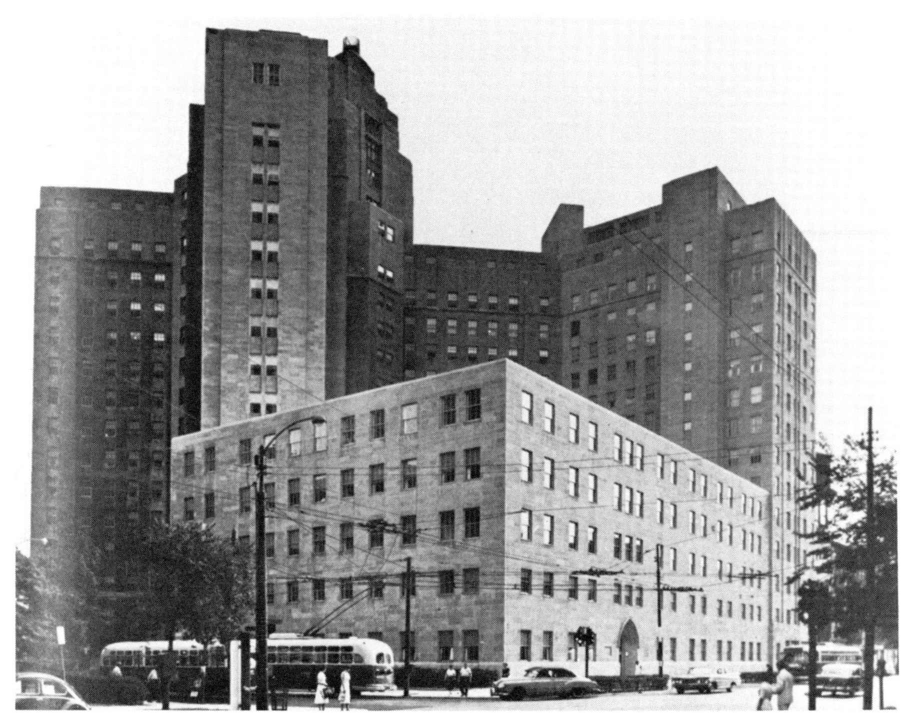

*Allison Pavilion, foreground, with doctors'
tower, rear right, was hailed "Hospital of
the future." For the first time in Chicago,
doctors' offices were built in a hospital.*

David R. Jaye completed his residency at Wesley and earned his master of science degree in hospital administration from Northwestern in 1953. He became an administrative assistant at Wesley and was assigned to the numerous details involved with the closure of Chicago Memorial Hospital and merger with Wesley.

Alan B. Campbell worked in Wesley's credit department while studying hospital administration at Northwestern. As administrative resident in 1954, he was in charge of the Hospital on Sundays. After receiving his degree he became administrator of Richland Memorial Hospital at Olney, Illinois.

Newell E. France, who had been graduated with honors and received his master of science degree in hospital administration from Northwestern, became Wesley's administrative assistant in charge of evening services in 1955. He resigned after a year to become assistant administrator of St. Luke's Episcopal Hospital at Houston, Texas.

In 1956 the job of administrative assistant in charge of evening service was assigned to *David L. Winebrenner*, who held a bachelor of arts degree from Wheaton College and his master's degree in hospital administration from Northwestern. His hospital residency was served at Brooke Army Hospital, Fort Sam Houston, San Antonio, Texas, following three years in army medical service in Korea and Japan. After a year at Wesley, Winebrenner was appointed director of personnel services.

Wesley's evening administrative assistant position was filled by *John A. Taft, Jr.* in 1957 after he had completed his hospital residency and earned his master's degree from Northwestern. Taft won an award from Alpha Delta Mu, professional fraternity in hospital administration, for the best paper submitted during the school year, entitled "Administrative Problems of Death and Autopsy."

PENSION PLAN BEGINS

Wesley's first pension plan became effective January 1, 1953, and the first employee to benefit was 80-year-old *Annie Morgan* who retired January 15. She had been employed at the age of 50 in 1923 as a "junior food service helper" in the dietary department and had performed those duties for 30 years. She explained to fellow employees at a department farewell party in her honor, "I'll keep busy with church work. No use sitting down and letting your bones get all stiff."

Fifteen employees who were over 65 and had worked many years at the Hospital were paid tribute by Wesley President Stiles at a tea April 30, 1954, on the occasion of their retirement. The honorees were: *Joseph Cohn*, service; *Mary Faherty*, nursing; *Louise Jones*, social service; *John Maloney*, service; *Ann Matthews*, nursing; *Jeanette Mitchell*, nursing; *Charles Nugara*, dietary; *Titus Palm*, maintenance; *Florence Rood*, housekeeping; *Coila Richards*, dietary; *Nettie Simen*, nursing education; *George Solas*, dietary; *Marie Tennis*, nursing; *Alice Thompson* and *Mabel Van Doren*, service.

Another "old timer" was *Andy Bloomberg*, a master craftsman and painter, who laid down his brushes and tools at the age of 70. He retired in May, 1954, with the enviable record of only six days' absence due to illness in 42 years of service at old and new Wesley. It was said that he could transform a decrepit chair, sofa or desk into furniture that looked like new.

Wesley nursing graduate *Minnie B. Howe*, Class of 1911, who had served as assistant nursing director in charge of evening duty for a quarter of a century, also retired in 1954. After receiving her diploma, she spent 18 years in supervisory and administrative positions in several hospitals, returning to Wesley in 1929. One veteran nurse recalled, "One could always count on Miss Howe's appearance on duty at 3 p.m. She had almost perfect attendance for 25 years." Kenath Hartman, then assistant to the superintendent, said, "I had heard and read of women who had given their lives to nursing. I had hoped that sometime during my career I would have the opportunity to meet such a rare woman. To me, Miss Howe will forever be identified with nursing, personifying Florence Nightingale's work."

Sena H. Brandt,[1] who retired as nursing arts instructor in 1954 spent much of her professional life at Wesley. A graduate of Wesley's Class of 1912, she worked for 12 years as a private duty nurse in the Chicago area, returning to Wesley in 1924 as educational director and nursing arts instructor. After ten years she moved to Iowa and became a hospital nursing director, returning to Wesley in 1943.

A 1914 graduate of Wesley's school of nursing, *Ida C. Deardorff*, R.N., R.R.L., retired in March, 1955, having served 42 years at Wesley. After receiving her diploma in nursing, she cared for Wesley patients as a private duty nurse for 15 years. She had been a charter member of the American

[1]*Miss Brandt was honored at a 1977 Wesley Nurse Alumnae reunion. She died in 1979 in her home at Elgin, Illinois at the age of 91.*

Association of Medical Record Librarians in 1929 and had become supervisor of Old Wesley's medical records department. She came to the new hospital as evening supervisor of the record room.

When *Katherine N. Williams*, social service director, retired in March, 1956, she probably had the longest association of any employee with Wesley. As a young girl she came from North Wales in 1906 to visit an aunt who had been one of the first patients admitted to Wesley when it was in a frame house on Ohio Street in 1888. Determined to be a nurse, Katherine made the rounds of nursing schools but all except Wesley turned her down because she was only 16. Within a month after graduation in 1909 she became a supervisor on the woman's surgical ward and eight months later joined the nursing school office as assistant supervisor until her marriage in 1913.

After the death of her husband in 1921 Mrs. Williams became a receptionist at Wesley's information desk until 1929 when she was placed in charge of social service. There her warmth and friendly efficiency helped thousands of patients during the next 27 years. Following retirement, Katherine Williams went to live with her daughter and son-in-law, Dr. J. Fred Merritt, a former Wesley intern practicing in Greensboro, North Carolina. Katherine's many friends at Wesley were saddened to learn of her death just one year later.

Mrs. Williams was succeeded as social service director by *Cleone Hansen*, a graduate of the Evanston School of Nursing. She had been director of nursing at South Shore Hospital and American Hospital, both in Chicago, before taking charge of Wesley's social service department.

A Well Received Announcement

The decade's happiest news of nurses came on June 28, 1958, at the annual banquet of the Wesley Nurses' Alumnae Association. Bertha L. Knapp, director of nursing service and the school of nursing from 1908 to 1943, rose to speak to the 200 graduates present and announced, "I'm going to be married." When applause subsided, she continued, "Sixty years ago a young man proposed to me. I almost said yes, but since I had just graduated from nursing school I decided to pursue my career and not marry immediately. Four years later he married someone else. Now, many years later, this man is alone and again has asked me to marry him. This time I said yes."

Bertha Knapp had received her diploma in nursing from the University of Michigan in 1898. The young man who proposed was Dr. Richard A. Smith, director of the university's geology department. The two had gone their separate ways with Dr. Smith becoming an important conservationist and Miss Knapp, as head of nursing at Wesley, an influential leader in her profession. She had never married. Miss Knapp, 79, and Dr. Smith, 81, were married July 24, 1958, at her summer home in Neillsville, Wisconsin.

Wesley Loses Eight Physicians

Dr. Raymond W. McNealy, chairman of Wesley's surgery department for 24 of his 31 years on the staff, died July 29, 1958, at the age of 71. He suffered a heart attack while attending a patient in his office at Wesley and succumbed half an hour later. He had graduated with highest honors in 1910 from the University of Illinois Medical School and had interned at Cook County Hospital in 1911 where, 20 years later, he became president of the staff, serving until his death. Only two weeks earlier he had announced his decision to retire as president of the Cook County staff January 1, "to make way for younger men," he said. He was chief of staff at Wesley in 1939 and 1940 and a member of the Board of Trustees for many years.

In the critical period between late 1939 and 1941, Dr. McNealy had suspended his medical practice temporarily to travel to other cities to accumulate information on efficient planning of hospital services to apply to the new building. He served as the superintendent of the Hospital in 1941, directing the move from Old Wesley. It was Dr. McNealy who arranged with the artist, John H. DeRosen, to paint the mural, *The Divine Healer,* symbolizing Wesley's service to humanity.

In his early days after receiving his M.D. degree, Dr. McNealy went to Europe to do postgraduate work at the University of Vienna. In 1949, he returned to Vienna to attend the opening of the Austrian chapter of the International College of Surgeons. He was arrested and held captive briefly by the Russians. According to the *Chicago Daily News* of July 30, 1938, he was shipped out of Vienna in a boxcar. He was president of the United

Research Foundation and chairman of the United States qualifications board of the international college.

Death claimed seven other members of the Wesley medical staff in the nineteen fifties. *Dr. Theodore T. Stone*, 54, chairman of Wesley's neuro-psychiatry department since 1943, died March 5, 1952, after a long illness. Dr. Stone received his M.D. degree from the University of Illinois in 1919, his M.S. degree in 1933 and Ph.D. degree in 1935 from Northwestern.

Dr. Garwood C. Richardson, member of Wesley's attending staff in obstetrics and gynecology for 20 years, died March 4, 1953, at Wesley following a heart attack. Dr. Richardson was graduated from Northwestern University Medical School in 1922.

Dr. Eugene B. Perry, assistant professor of urology at Northwestern and member of Wesley's attending staff since 1922, died May 11, 1953, at the age of 60. Born in Melvin, Illinois, he had served as a first lieutenant in the medical corps during World War I before moving to Chicago in 1923. He received his medical education at Rush Medical College and Brady Urological Institute of Johns Hopkins University.

Dr. Mark T. Goldstine, 75, who had joined Wesley in 1902 when the Hospital was 14 years old, died March 4, 1954, of a stroke during a motor trip in Georgia. He was a graduate of Rush Medical College, spent two years in practice and research at Rotunda Hospital in Dublin, Ireland, and joined the Northwestern faculty in 1911. Dr. Goldstine distinguished himself in obstetrics and gynecology and he was active in cancer research for almost 40 years. In 1915 he established and personally maintained a cancer clinic at Wesley. In 1936 the Davella Mills Foundation offered financial assistance to cancer research at Wesley and named Dr. Goldstine director of the work.

Dr. Nathan Smith Davis III, 66, who had joined the Wesley staff and Northwestern faculty in 1921, died April 20, 1955, following a heart attack. Dr. Davis was a graduate of Harvard University and received his medical degree from Rush Medical College. His father and grandfather had been distinguished physicians, nationally known for reforms in medical education and active in the early progress of Northwestern University Medical School and Wesley Hospital.

Dr. James R. Webster, 51, well-known dermatologist and member of Wesley's senior staff, died February 21, 1958, after a long respiratory illness. He was a diplomate of the American Board of Dermatology and Syphilology, was president (1957) of the American Academy of Dermatology and Syphilology and a past president of the Chicago Dermatological Association.

Dr. Emery G. Grimm, 64, endocrinologist, member of the Wesley medical staff and Northwestern faculty for 16 years, died March 19, 1959. Born in Hungary, he studied at the University of Budapest and graduated in 1921 from the University of Vienna, then spent a year as instructor in internal medicine in Budapest. He came to the United States in 1923 and made five subsequent European trips for postgraduate work at two universities. His research interests included studies of the relationship between ductless glands and obesity, and the failure of some children to grow normally.

RALPH HUESTON RETIRES

The year 1959 ended with the announcement that Ralph M. Hueston would retire January 15, 1960, after 12 years as superintendent. When he joined the Hospital in 1948, its properties consisted of New Wesley, the old building and Hampshire House. Under his leadership the Hospital grew and expanded its services considerably. Old Wesley was sold and properties at 226 and 230 East Superior were acquired. Property at 228 East Superior Street was purchased, consolidating holdings immediately west of Wesley into one piece with a frontage of eighty feet. Wesley further increased its assets when it merged with Chicago Memorial Hospital and became Chicago Wesley Memorial Hospital in 1954. By the end of the decade, the Allison Pavilion was in full operation and the Cathedral of Healing had been extensively remodeled. Mr. Hueston was active in hospital and allied organizations, serving as president of the Chicago Hospital Council and of the National Association of Hospitals and Homes of the Methodist Church. He was a member of the Board of Directors of the Community Hospital of Evanston, the Illinois Hospital Association, Hospital Service Corporation (Blue Cross for Illinois), Illinois League for Nursing and the Methodist Old Peoples Home.

Consolidating Resources 1960 to September, 1972

Part IV

The Restless Sixties Chapter 20

Turbulence and unrest spread throughout the nation during Wesley's seventh decade, its third on Northwestern's near north Chicago campus. At the Hospital, however, 1960 began on a quiet note of confidence indicative of a new but capable administration, a first-rate medical staff, modern facilities and financial solvency.

At the annual meeting of the Board of Trustees on January 9, Kenath Hartman, assistant to the retiring superintendent Ralph M. Hueston for the past twelve years, was elected superintendent. He was a graduate of Washington University in St. Louis, Missouri, and held a master's degree in hospital administration from Northwestern University. He was a coordinator and lecturer for the Northwestern course and a fellow of the American College of Hospital Administrators.

Donald A. Bloom, another graduate of Northwestern's hospital administration course, had been employed as comptroller at Wesley in 1948 and was advanced to assistant superintendent and comptroller in 1960. A decided advantage to patients and the Hospital was the introduction of IBM procedures in handling admissions, billings and payment of bills. Under comptroller Bloom's supervision, the IBM system already had reduced the work load in various departments and business personnel had been decreased while production was accelerated.

Another new system benefiting patients, physicians and employees was silent electronic paging. This method eliminated up to 100 public address page calls per hour that formerly were heard throughout Wesley over the old paging system. The new program provided pocket-sized transistor radios for all attending physicians, house staff and key personnel who moved about the hospital. Doctors with their "beepers" could be contacted within a two-mile radius whether the recipient was at Passavant Hospital, Veterans Hospital or Northwestern Medical School.

REINFORCING ORGANIZATION

The Board of Trustees had taken several steps to strengthen the professional organization. President Arthur Dole, Jr., reported, "We have restated the objectives of the Hospital in terms of its being a teaching and research unit of Northwestern University. We have strengthened the lines of communication between the trustees, the medical staff, the hospital administration and Northwestern University by making the liaison committee a standing committee of the Board of Trustees. We now invite the chief of the medical staff and an alternate to attend the meetings of the Board of Trustees." Accordingly, Chief of Staff Edward M. Dorr gave his report at the 1960 meeting and predicted that the board's action would improve both communications and the teaching program. Dr. Dorr, obstetrician and gynecologist, had succeeded Dr. Joseph F. Mallach as chief of staff.

The appointment of Dr. David P. Earle, professor of medicine at Northwestern, as chairman of Wesley's new department of research in 1960 further strengthened the professional organization. Dr. Earle was a graduate of Princeton University and the College of Physicians and Surgeons at Columbia University. In 1954 he had joined the Northwestern faculty and the Passavant staff where he was principal investigator for research grants of more than ten million dollars to the two institutions from the National Institutes of Health.

EXTENDING RESEARCH

Research at Wesley had increased so rapidly that recently constructed facilities were inadequate by 1960. Application for funds for additional laboratories were made to the National Institutes of Health. Among the projects under way in the 34 laboratories then available were:

Tissue Culture Laboratory Pioneer observations on the development of the ear. Studies in bone formation and effects of noxious agents on the function of respiratory cells.

Surgical Research Laboratory Studies of the development of artificial aortic valves, a new capillary membrane oxygenator and the evaluation of chemotherapeutic agents on cancer cell suspensions.

Neurosurgical Research Laboratory Studies on the effects of various central nervous system lesions on muscular activity and psychological behavior in monkeys.

Urological Research Laboratory Observations on hormone metabolism during the course of treatment of prostatic cancer.

The application was approved by the NIH and work began at once on expanded research laboratories in the Ruth Jones Allison Pavilion. They were opened June 12, 1962, and included four laboratories for surgical and steroid hormonal research, a clinical isotope research laboratory, an automatic amino acid analyzer laboratory, an animal research room, small animal quarters, a low temperature laboratory and four research offices. The cost of $200,965 was provided by the NIH, the Schweppe Foundation and the Wesley Service League.

The NIH also approved a grant to Northwestern University for cardiovascular research conducted at Wesley. The grant supported not only the work of Dr. Paul Kezdi, heart station director, and his associates, but efforts of other departments also helping heart patients. These included the pharmacology department which examined the action of new drugs on the cardiovascular system, the surgical department where new artificial valves and their function were being studied, and Northwestern's Technological Institute where electronic equipment for diagnosis and control of cardiovascular disease was being developed.

COORDINATING TEACHING AND RESEARCH

The medical teaching program was reorganized by Dr. Thomas C. Laipply, director of medical services, which included medical education. He helped develop a coordinated program of research and education, creating renewed interest among staff members. For the first time in years Wesley obtained its full quota of 26 interns and 56 residents plus two fellows in neuro-psychiatry and one in orthopedics. The increased house staff posed a dwelling problem which was alleviated by the purchase of a building with 82 apartments at 180 East Delaware Place. The transaction was financed by bank loans and sale of the 36-apartment building at 222 East Delaware.

In another area of education, the School of Nursing, the Wesley board concurred with a recommendation of its committee on nursing to discontinue the four-year degree program offered in conjunction with Northwestern University. In September, 1960, the full quota of 110 students entered the three-year course in nursing. In the fall of the following year, Wesley's payroll had 174 staff nurses, the highest number ever at that time of year. However, hospital occupancy was so great that the ratio between nurses and patients was not as high as in previous years. This was a trend that would reach dangerous proportions in thousands of hospitals before the end of the decade.

EMPHASIS ON NURSING

In an effort to curtail the effects of a nurse shortage, Wesley took steps in January, 1963, to increase the efficiency of the nursing department. Virginia R. Keller was employed as the Hospital's first full-time nurse to coordinate the inservice education program for professional staff nurses and auxiliary personnel. She also arranged refresher courses for professional nurses who had not practiced for several years. Need for continued nurse education was shown by the fact that 90 percent of the drugs used in 1963 were unknown in 1953. Mrs. Keller held a master's degree in education from Loyola University and had been employed in nursing education at Presbyterian-St. Luke's, Little Company of Mary, and Passavant hospitals.

E. Elizabeth Geiger, Wesley nursing director for nine years, retired in July, 1963, and Emma L. Grimm was appointed acting director of nursing service. She had been on the nursing administration staff of Old Wesley and had helped organize the department of the new hospital in 1941. Lois Ebinher was named acting director of nursing education.

Across the country the nurse shortage was becoming critical for hospitals as industry, transportation, government and highly endowed medical centers siphoned off available nurses. At Wesley the situation was serious even though 22 of the 39 graduates of the Class of 1964 elected to remain. For the first time patient occupancy averaged 90 percent for the entire year.

FORMER NAVY COMMANDER HEADS NURSING SERVICE

A recently retired commander in the U.S. Navy Nurse Corps, Vera Eileen Thompson, was appointed director of nursing at Wesley effective May 1, 1964. A native Pennsylvanian, she was a graduate of Williamsport Hospital School of Nursing, had earned a B.S. degree in medical-surgical nursing from Columbia University and held a master's degree in counseling from George Washington University. At the outbreak of World War II, she enlisted in the Navy Nurse Corps and was commissioned an ensign.

The war years took Mrs. Thompson to naval hospitals at Bethesda, Maryland; Oakland, California; Philadelphia, as well as base hospitals in Finchhafen, New Guinea, and Manus in the Admiralty Isles. She was commissioned a commander in 1957 while education officer for the nursing division of the Bureau of Medicine and Surgery, Department of Navy. Later she was coordinator of nursing service of the 600-bed navy hospital at San Diego, California.

PREPARED FOR ACTION

In the spring of 1961 the medical staff arranged a practice drill of Wesley's revised catastrophe plan directed by Dr. T. Howard Clarke. The "dry run" was thwarted, however, when, at 10:20 p.m. March 24, an explosion ripped through a tavern basement on Wells Street, about three-fourths of a mile from Wesley. The cause of the blast was unknown, but police suspected a bomb.

The maximum force of the explosion was just beneath the tavern floor where guests were dancing. A number of them fell into the basement through a gaping hole torn in the floor. About 40 persons were injured from flying glass and debris, or the fall into the basement. Of the total, 25 casualties were rushed to Wesley, the largest number to be treated simultaneously in Wesley's emergency department on the Northwestern campus.

With calm efficiency, Wesley doctors, nurses and administrative personnel quickly went into action. Interns, residents and attending physicians answered the emergency call promptly. Doctors and nurses as well as laboratory, blood bank and anesthesia personnel all coordinated their responsibilities according to the plan. Five of the Wesley patients were critically injured and the others had minor cuts and bruises. Of the most seriously injured, one woman underwent amputation of both legs and her right arm; a second woman lost both legs.

Unquestionably, one of the reasons for the efficient action was the advance planning for just such an emergency by the Catastrophe Committee of the Medical Staff. Their competent performance was praised by the Red Cross disaster crew, the police and the press.

All together, 20,574 emergency patients were treated in 1961. During the year, 18,077 patients (an increase of 687 over the previous year) were admitted to Wesley's 657 beds. In 1962, Dr. Durand Smith, newly elected chief of staff, in his report to the trustees, said "The high census has made it difficult to admit patients on scheduled days in spite of the recently adopted policy for controlling the number of admissions accepted for any one day."

A popular new facility opened at that time was a seven-bed diagnostic unit for patients admitted by their attending physician, but who required minimal or no nursing care. The attractive accommodations and services were frequently used by business executives desiring annual intensive medical check-ups.

HARWOOD BECOMES PRESIDENT

Thomas A. Harwood, president of George Fry & Associates, consulting management engineers, and Wesley trustee for 21 years, was elected president at the 1961 annual meeting of the Wesley Board of Trustees. He succeeded Arthur Dole, Jr., who had served since 1958. Harwood's consultant background had been particularly valuable to the budget committee which he had chaired since 1943. As a Northwestern University graduate and past president of the Alumni Association, he was keenly aware of the bond that linked Wesley Hospital and the Northwestern Medical School.

TRUSTEES OF THE SIXTIES

Board members elected early in the decade were particularly well qualified to deal with problems peculiar to the period in which they served. *Henry E.*

Seyfarth, partner in the law firm of Seyfarth, Shaw, Fairweather and Geraldson, was elected to the Wesley board in 1960. He was board chairman of both the Union National Bank of Chicago and the First National Bank of Blue Island and on the board of several charitable and civic organizations, including the Urban League. In the same year, *Rawleigh Warner*, chairman of the board of The Pure Oil Company, also was elected a Wesley trustee. A graduate of Princeton University, he was a director of American Petroleum Institute, the City National Bank and Trust Company of Chicago and the International Minerals and Chemicals Corporation. In World War II he had served as a special assistant to the Secretary of the Navy and as chairman of the Navy's Procurement Review Board, receiving the Distinguished Civilian Service Award.

T. Stanton Armour, partner in the investment firm of Mitchell, Hutchins & Company, joined the Wesley board in 1961. He was a member of the Chicago Board of Trade and the Midwest Stock Exchange, and a director of the Chicago Salvation Army. During the following year the Wesley board added four members: *A. Newell Rumpf*, senior vice president of Harris Trust & Savings Bank of Chicago; *William Wrigley*, president of the William Wrigley Jr. Company and a director of Wrigley companies in seven countries; *Hubert E. Howard, Jr.*, vice president of Shaster Coal Corporation; and *Donald M. Graham*, vice chairman of the Continental-Illinois National Bank & Trust Company of Chicago. Clergymen joining the board in the early sixties were *Dr. Harold A. Bosley*, minister of the First Methodist Church of Evanston, and *Dr. Robert Bruce Pierce*, minister of the Chicago Temple, the First Methodist Church of Chicago.

Marguerite Stitt Church, who had retired voluntarily from the Congress of the United States after 12 years of service, was elected to the Wesley Board of Trustees in 1963. Following graduation from Wellesley College, she received an LL.D degree from Russell Sage College in Troy, New York, and honorary doctorates in law from Lake Forest College and Northwestern University. Among her many appointments were United States delegate to the General Assembly of the United Nations, 1961, and later, a member of the planning board for the White House Conference on Aging.

Mrs. Church became the third woman on the Wesley board at that time. *Mrs. (Marion) Stanley B. Zaring*, daughter of George W. Dixon, former

Wesley president, had been elected a trustee in 1956, joining her aunt, *Mrs. (Edna) Paul Walker*, daughter of Arthur Dixon, the original Dixon trustee. Edna Dixon Walker was an active board member from 1929 until 1962 when she became an emeritus trustee.

SPREADING KNOWLEDGE AROUND THE WORLD

The honors bestowed on Wesley medical staff members verified excellence in their specialties and evidenced quality of care in the Hospital where the work was conducted. The physicians were teaching at home and abroad to disseminate knowledge originating at Wesley. The following items were gleaned from various Wesley publications from 1961 through 1964. They represent but a scant sampling of the local, regional, national and international tributes received by Wesley physicians; many were honored before and after that period.

1961—*Dr. George E. Shambaugh, Jr.*, otolaryngologist, was elected president of the section on otolaryngology of the International College for Surgery of Deafness; at Paris he addressed the 7th International Congress for Otolaryngology. *Dr. Orion H. Stuteville*, otolaryngology, was elected president of the American Society of Maxillofacial Surgeons. He presented a paper on "Lesions of the Oral Cavity" at a seminar in Hawaii.

Dr. Benjamin Boshes, chairman of the departments of neurology and psychiatry at Wesley and Northwestern, was elected secretary for the United States to the World Federation of Neurology. On a trip to Greece, Turkey and Israel, he lectured on the physiology of spinal cord and Parkinson's disease at Hadassah Medical School in Jerusalem. *Dr. Paul C. Bucy*, chief of the neurosurgery section of Wesley's surgery department and president of the International Congress of Neurological Surgery meeting in Germany, received the Fedor Krause Commemorative Medal. Dr. Bucy was appointed to the Advisory Council of the National Institute of Neurological Diseases and Blindness, one of the U.S. National Institutes of Health. *Dr. Eloise E. Johnson*, pediatrics, addressed the 10th Rheumatological Congress in Rome.

Dr. Edward L. Compere, chairman of the Wesley department of orthopedics, addressed the 13th Biennial World Congress of the International College of Surgeons in New York on "Multiple Fractures of the Femur." *Dr. Clinton L. Compere*, orthopedics, was elected president of the American

Academy of Orthopaedic Surgeons. *Dr. John J. Bergan*, surgery, with *Dr. Marion C. Anderson* of Passavant, was awarded a gold medal citation from the Illinois State Medical Society and was cited by the American Medical Association for a scientific exhibit titled, "Significance of Vascular Injury in Pancreatitis."

1962—*Dr. Paul S. Rhoads*, chairman of the department of medicine at Wesley, was invited to India to assist the Ludhiana Medical College in reorganization. The school, supported by Methodist and Presbyterian churches in England, had a long and heroic history. *Dr. J. Kenneth Sokol*, urology, moderated a section on urological movies at the American College of Surgeons meeting in San Francisco. Included was the movie, "Left Brachial Angiography," produced at Wesley by *Drs. William G. Karras, Abram H. Cannon, J. Kenneth Sokol* and *Vincent J. O'Conor, Jr.*

Dr. Jacques M. Smith, medicine, was elected chief of staff of the Rehabilitation Institute of Chicago. *Dr. Durand Smith*, surgery, was recipient of the A. B. Graham Award from the American Proctologic Society for the best report of investigative work on non-malignant ulcerative diseases of the colon. *Dr. Vincent J. O'Conor, Jr.*, urology, gave the Bowman Gray Lecture on prediction methods in renal hypertension at Bowman Gray Medical School in Winston-Salem, North Carolina.

1963—*Dr. George H. Gardner*, chairman of the Wesley department of obstetrics and gynecology, was elected president of the American Gynecological Society. *Dr. Edward M. Dorr*, gynecology, was elected president of the American Association for Maternal and Infant Health.

Dr. Ture O. Tuncbay, neurology resident at Wesley, won the S. Weir Mitchell Award of the American Academy of Neurology, the highest honor accorded a medical trainee in the United States or Canada. Dr. Tuncbay, a native of Turkey and graduate of the University of Istanbul, was the first woman to win the prize. *Dr. Joel Brumlik* of the attending staff had won the award in 1961, making the Wesley research program the first to have two winners.

Dr. John L. Reichert, chairman of the Wesley department of pediatrics, chairman of the AMA's joint committee on health problems in education, was panel chairman on school health problems at the National Education Association meeting in Seattle. He received the George Howell Coleman Award given annually by the Institute of Medicine.

1964—*Dr. Roland P. Mackay*, neurology, presented the history of neurology in the Midwest before the Mayo Clinic Neurology Alumni Reunion at Rochester, and at the International College of Surgeons meeting.

Dr. Richard A. Perritt, ophthalmology, completed a 30,000-mile summer operating and lecture tour. In Manila he operated at Santo Thomas University, then flew to Singapore, Brisbane and Melbourne where, as official representative of the AMA, he lectured on micro-ophthalmic surgery at the Second Congress of the Asia-Pacific Academy of Ophthalmology. Earlier he was awarded the Honor Banner by the Free China Chapter of Ophthalmology in Formosa. In Europe he examined the eyes of Cardinal Alfredo Ottaviani, head of the Vatican's Holy Office, and of President Eamon de Valera of Ireland.

At the request of the Academy of Sciences of the USSR, *Dr. Hampar Kelikian*, orthopedics, lectured and performed hand surgery at Erevan, Moscow, Leningrad and the American University Hospital in Beirut, Lebanon, his native country. Dr. Kelikian received high praise in the March 22, 1964 issue of the *Chicago Tribune* for surgery performed on Congressman Robert Dole (now Senator) repairing injuries from a bomb in World War II. A three-column article described the series of operations in Wesley where Dr. Kelikian had transplanted bone, muscle and skin from Dole's leg to his shattered right shoulder, arm and hand, partially restoring their use and enabling him to continue a successful political career.

Death Claims Physicians and Trustees

For Wesley's active medical staff and board members, the exciting decade promised ample opportunity for service. For others whose missions had been fulfilled, it brought the satisfaction of having accepted challenges and successfully carried them through. Wesley mourned the loss of several dedicated friends and associates in the early 1960s.

1960—*George B. McKibbin*, 72, prominent attorney, Republican leader and Wesley trustee for 15 years, died September 15. He was state director of finance, 1941 to 1945, leaving the position briefly in 1943 to campaign as Republican candidate for mayor of Chicago. He was defeated by the incumbent, Mayor Edward J. Kelly.

Dr. Herman Chor, 56, neuropsychiatrist, died November 4. A graduate of Johns Hopkins University, he received his medical degree from the

University of Maryland, was a fellow in neurology at Mayo Clinic, and received a master of science degree from Northwestern. During World War II he was chief of neuropsychiatry at the Naval Base Hospital at Pearl Harbor.

1961—*Jay Lyman Hench*, 76, Wesley trustee for 20 years and president from 1948-1953, one of Wesley's outstanding leaders , died April 16. The son of a country doctor, he was born in Hinsdale, spent two years at Cornell University where he studied metallurgy, worked as a laborer, held several jobs before acquiring Mid-West Forging and Manufacturing Company, later becoming president. He was chairman of Wesley's budget committee from 1942 until 1948, during which time he established sound budgetary procedures and stabilized Wesley's financial position. A crowning achievement was the completion ten years ahead of schedule of payments on an $800,000 loan from Connecticut Mutual Life Insurance Company. The loan had been negotiated in 1941 to equip the new building.

John Holmes, Wesley trustee from 1942 until his death October 21, 1961, had had the unique experience of being president before attending a board meeting. His predecessor, Thomas J. Thomas, had served only three months in late 1941 when he was called to Washington for government war service. Holmes, president of Swift & Company, took leadership when Wesley was struggling to meet wartime obligations with critically inadequate working capital. John Holmes arrived in the United States from Belfast, Ireland, and rose from messenger boy to president of one of the nation's largest companies, in accord with the best American tradition.

1962—Within four weeks, Wesley lost four members of its senior attending staff. *Dr. David E. Markson*, 74, specialist in rheumatic diseases and 1912 medical graduate of Northwestern, died March 6 in Downey Veterans Hospital. *Dr. Arthur E. Mahle*, 68, specialist in internal medicine, chief of staff at Wesley from 1956 to 1958, and medical director of the Old Peoples Home in Chicago, died at his home March 26. On the same day, *Dr. Hayden E. E. Barnard*, 65, surgeon and head of surgical anatomy at Northwestern University from 1925 to 1935, died at Wesley. He was a 1918 graduate of Rush Medical College. *Dr. Francis D. Wolfe*, 61, proctology specialist, Northwestern medical graduate of 1927, died unexpectedly at his home April 1.

Dr. Walter Grierson Maddock, 60, chairman of the Wesley department of surgery since 1952, died at Wesley on October 26. He was a founding member of the American Board of Surgery and recipient of the Distinguished Service Award of the American Cancer Society in 1961. In World War II he was an army colonel and commanding officer of the 298th general hospital, receiving the Legion of Merit.

1963—*Dr. Vincent John O'Conor*, 69, chairman of Wesley's department of urology, died at his home January 26 after attending the annual meeting of the medical staff at the University Club earlier in the evening. He was a graduate of Rush Medical College, served an internship at Presbyterian Hospital and a urological residency at Peter Bent Brigham Hospital in Boston. Dr. O'Conor came to Wesley in 1942 from the Washington Boulevard Hospital. He was Wesley chief of staff from 1948 to 1950 and Northwestern chairman of urology from 1947 to 1961. He had been president of the American Association of Genito-Urinary Surgeons.

Dr. Arthur Metz, 76, surgeon, had a heart attack on a train en route to New York, and returned by ambulance from Plymouth, Indiana to Wesley where he died June 15. He was a graduate of Indiana University in 1909 and of Rush Medical College in 1911. Dr. Metz was chief of staff at Wahington Boulevard Hospital until it closed in 1942, when he joined the Wesley staff. In 1953 he received Indiana University's distinguished alumni service award. He was a commodore of the Chicago Yacht Club.

1964—*Dr. John L. Reichert*, Wesley pediatrician since 1952, died of a heart attack in his office September 19. He was on the courtesy staffs of Children's Memorial and Evanston hospitals, and a leader in child health protection in the Chicago area for 41 years. Shortly before his death he received the George Howell Coleman Award.

Dr. Edward M. Dorr, obstetrics, suffered a heart attack in his home October 25. He came to Wesley in 1947 and twice served as chief of staff. He was president of the American Association of Maternal and Child Health at the time of his death.

PRESIDENT HARWOOD DIES

Thomas A. Harwood, president of the Wesley Board of Trustees since 1961 and member since 1940, died January 27, 1964, after a brief illness. He was president of the consultant firm, George Fry & Associates, and his far-sighted business acumen had helped Wesley weather the depression, complete and open the building on Northwestern's campus and construct the Allison Pavilion. A 1915 Northwestern graduate, he served on the Northwestern-Wesley relations committee, was past president of the N. U. Alumni Association and the N. U. Club of Chicago. He had enlisted in the field artillery in World War I and at war's end he was a first lieutenant.

Before his death, Mr. Harwood had established a trust with Wesley as the sole beneficiary. Wesley trustees later voted to use the funds to establish an intensive care unit as a memorial to Thomas A. Harwood.

WILLIAM ALEXANDER NAMED SUCCESSOR

William Henry Alexander, secretary of the Wesley Board of Trustees, since 1956, was elected vice president and named acting president of the board immediately after the death of Thomas Harwood. At a board meeting the following June 8, Mr. Alexander was elected president. He was a partner in the law firm of Ashcraft, Olson, Beach, Alexander and Edmonds and a former president of the Chicago Bar Association. He had joined the Wesley board in 1954 and was a trustee of Northwestern University.

Samuel W. Witwer, partner in the law firm of Witwer, Moran & Burlage, and Wesley trustee since 1951, was elected to the vacated office of secretary. At the same meeting in June the board elected two new trustees: Milburn P. Akers, editor of the *Sun-Times*, and Roscoe G. Haynie, chief executive officer of Wilson and Co., meat packing company.

DR. O'CONOR, JR., UROLOGY CHAIRMAN

Dr. Vincent J. O'Conor, Jr. was appointed chairman of the department of urology June 1, 1963, succeeding his father who had died in January. A native of Chicago, Dr. O'Conor was graduated from Yale University, cum laude from Northwestern University Medical School, and took his surgical training at Peter Bent Brigham Hospital in Boston where he was a member of the team initiating kidney transplantation. He had been on the Northwestern faculty since 1950, and was attending urologist at the V. A. Research Hospital and the Rehabilitation Institute of Chicago. He participated in cooperative studies of the National Institutes of Health relating to renovascular hypertension.

Planning Ahead   Chapter 21

Nearly every Wesley statistic was surpassed in the year 1965 when 21,212 patients occupied the Hospital's 700 beds. Newborn babies numbered 1,985 and emergency treatment was given to 23,478 persons. Bringing care and comfort to patients were 205 doctors, 63 residents, 33 interns, 34 medical students serving as clerks, and 1,550 employees including 230 registered nurses. Wesley personnel records listed over 300 job categories, making most employees specialists in their own sphere.

Increased grants supported additional research and service which, in turn, required more workers, sometimes hastily hired to meet critical needs. One by-product of this rapid growth was definitely detrimental: slack security. Hospital equipment and supplies escaped through unguarded doors and a rash of petty thievery plagued patients, personnel and visitors.

SOLVING THE SECURITY PROBLEM

Following newspaper reports of two Wesley employees arrested with stolen hospital property, the trustees authorized a security survey to be conducted by the Pinkerton Detective Agency.

A five-point program was recommended and Russell L. Colling, who had completed a similar assignment at Memorial Hospital of DuPage County in Elmhurst, was employed to implement it. The requirements were: (1)

Identification badges for all personnel. (2) Fingerprinting and photographing all employees. (3) Identification of packages carried by employees leaving the hospital. (4) Adequate security personnel to investigate all thefts or other security incidents occurring within the hospital premises. (5) Use of electronic means of maintaining security.

The measures were planned to end thievery, minimize misuse of equipment and materials and safeguard employees in and near the Hospital. Fingerprinting and photographing of all hospital employees began in January, 1965. A closed circuit television was installed in the Northwestern University tunnel which relayed a constant picture to the Central Security Center in Wesley. Three mirrors in hallways near the center gave uniformed officers a clear view of all activity near the employee exit.

Colling, who held a B.S. degree in police administration from Michigan State University, had selected 18 thoroughly screened men who were given 30 hours of intense training before going on duty. In addition, the officers attended weekly classes conducted by the Chicago Police Force Academy at Michael Reese Hospital.

The area between Wesley and its residences where persons had been accosted at night was under constant evening surveillance. Officers with walkie-talkies patrolled the vicinity and provided escort service between 11 p.m. and 1:15 a.m. for nurses and students individually or in groups. The security men made nightly checks of all of Wesley's properties. Internal pilfering of food, linens and other supplies was controlled by limiting employee entrances and exits to two doors and by checking packages.

So effective was Wesley's security program that three years later it was acclaimed first among all institutional security programs in the United States and Canada by the International Security Conference in 1968.

WESLEY AND PUBLIC RELATIONS
From its beginning, Wesley had been on friendly terms with the communications media, which usually reported Hospital events in a favorable light. After World War II, public interest in health care issues created a need for hospital communications specialists to act as liaisons with the media, provide accurate information to the press, prepare publications for particular readership[1], handle special events and direct fund raising. These services

[1]*Patients, visitors, employees, nurses, doctors, volunteers and the community at large*

had developed into an administrative department called *public relations* or *public information*. The Reverend Thaddeus Allen handled public relations duties at Wesley from the time it moved to its new building in 1941 through 1943, when a PR consultant firm was engaged.

The first journalist to be employed at Wesley as public relations director, a position established in 1949, was David J. Atchison, former newspaper editor, war correspondent, and assistant public relations director of the American Medical Association. At Wesley he handled press queries, edited publications and performed other services of the new specialty.

John R. Kinsey, a former newspaper man, succeeded Atchison in 1951. Under Kinsey's direction, *Wesley MEMO* for employees, *Wesley Life* for friends outside and the *Annual Report* continued to enlighten Wesley's special publics, and the good rapport between Hospital and media assured community support. Wesley publications won seven consecutive first place awards between 1953 and 1959 in the annual national MacEachern Competition[1] for hospital publications sponsored by *Hospital Management* magazine. Kinsey resigned in November, 1961, to become public information director of the American Hospital Association. He was replaced by John C. Erwin, also a journalist and public relations man who died of heart disease in 1963 at age 43. Continuity was provided to the department by the public relations assistant, Marjorie W. Roelle, who had joined the department in 1956. Her capable handling of information, contacts and records smoothed the way for the effective functioning of the department.

Arnie F. Betts came to Wesley in November, 1963, as director of publications and public information. A graduate of the University of Wisconsin School of Journalism, Betts had worked for Wisconsin newspapers and was on the development and public relations staff of the Illinois Institute of Technology. His editorial talent produced publications that dramatically portrayed medical achievements within Wesley. His knack in media relations was evident in articles appearing in local and national newspapers and magazines. A seven-page feature article on Wesley's radiology department appeared in the June, 1964, issue of *Look* magazine.

Another life-saving service at Wesley was publicized the next month in a July issue of the *Chicago's American,* Sunday supplement, a syndicated

[1]*In 1969, sponsorship of the 25-year-old MacEachern Competition was assumed by the Academy of Hospital Public Relations, founded in 1964.*

section which carried an article and photos showing a medical team from Wesley resuscitating a victim of cardiac arrest.

Who was John Wesley?

After 75 years of operation, the Hospital finally obtained a painting of its namesake, the great religious leader and physician John Wesley. The oil painting, *John Wesley, The Healer,* was purchased by the Woman's Auxiliary in memory of the recently deceased Thomas A. Harwood, president of the board. Evanston artist John R. White painted the subject from earlier likenesses on a three-by-four-foot canvas hung in the east corridor of the first floor April 8, 1964. John Wesley was shown with a nurse giving aid to sick children in the free dispensary he had opened in Bristol, in 1746. The legend on brass plates above and below the painting told part of the story of the physician-founder of Methodism.

John Wesley had completed his studies of medicine and theology at Lincoln College, Oxford, and was ordained a priest in the Church of England in 1728. He preached in towns near his birthplace, Epworth, Lincolnshire, until 1735 when he and his younger brother, Charles, accompanied James Oglethorpe to the colony, Georgia, John as a missionary and Charles as secretary to Oglethorpe, administrator of the colony. John returned to England in less than two years and continued his evangelistic work. He is said to have traveled about 250,000 miles, mostly on horseback, while preaching some 40,000 sermons.[1]

Wesley, the Healer

John Wesley combined his religious work with medicine, and he opened free dispensaries throughout England, gaining a considerable reputation as a physician. He wrote a number of books on healing and his *Easy and Natural Way of Curing Most Diseases* was the accepted English family medicine book through 23 editions. He was said to be the "greatest health educator of the 18th Century in Britain." John Wesley was one of the few college-educated physicians of his day.[2]

Before the painting was unveiled at Wesley it had received nationwide exposure. The Hospital and the Woman's Auxiliary granted *Together* magazine the rights to publish it as the double-fold full-color cover for its

[1]*The Columbia Encyclopedia, second edition*
[2]*Ibid*

February, 1964 issue. *Together*, Methodist Church family magazine, had a readership of 2,500,000 people.

MULTI-GIFTED HOSPITAL VOLUNTEERS

Wesley's five women's groups—Woman's Auxiliary, Service League, Volunteers, Patients' Library and Nurses Alumnae—had been organized in 1960 into the Wesley Volunteer Council, with each pursuing its original purpose, but with overall coordination. The council gave an annual Volunteer Service Award dinner where volunteers received gold pins for 1,000 hours of service, and a pearl for each additional 1,000 hours.

The next year Council members joined Sears Roebuck and Co. in a spectacular two-day show presenting fashions from Sears' 75-year history. First, Wesley volunteers boarded an Eastern Air Lines super electra and modeled clothes for fashion writers as the plane flew over North Redwood, Minnesota, the small town where Sears was founded in 1886, two years before the founding of Wesley. A repeat performance at the Pick-Congress Hotel the next day attracted hundreds of hospital friends.

In 1965 the Wesley Service League sponsored a show at the Chicago Amphitheatre that raised $25,000 for nuclear research. The world-famous Royal Marine Tattoo, official bandsmen for British marines, entertained a huge audience with two military bands, bag pipers, Scots guards, Highland dancers and the Royal Marines Motorcycle Drill Squad. Mrs. George Dixon, Jr., was chairman of the event.

VOLUNTEER OF THE YEAR

Each year Wesley selected a "Volunteer of the Year" as a candidate for the city-wide contest sponsored by the Volunteer Bureau of the Welfare Council of Metropolitan Chicago. Wesley's choice for 1965 was Dorothy Blott, whose 4,500 hours of service had been spent doing virtually every volunteer duty in the Hospital. A licensed practical nurse when she came to Wesley in 1944 as a Red Cross volunteer, Dorothy Blott had recruited and trained countless volunteers in nurses' aide procedures. She had wrapped bandages, lectured church groups and been in the forefront of every volunteer innovation from admitting office participation to the recovery room hostess program.

Two dedicated women had served as director of volunteers since Agnes

Spangler retired in 1961 after nearly five years of service. She was replaced by Ruth B. Webster, former director of volunteers at Cook County Hospital, and widow of Dr. James R. Webster, well-known Wesley dermatologist. She had long been a member of the Wesley Service League, which was organized by doctors' wives, and had served a two-year term as president.

Mrs. Webster resigned in 1963 and was succeeded by Elizabeth Greene, graduate of St. Luke's Hospital school of nursing and wife of Dr. Ronald R. Greene of Wesley's obstetrics and gynecology department. She also had been president of the Wesley Service League. When Mrs. Greene resigned in May, 1965, Wesley's volunteer of the year, Dorothy Blott, accepted the job until a new director came on the scene.

In September, Elizabeth Drees, chairman of the board of Newberry Center Settlement House, became Wesley's director of volunteers. She was the widow of the Reverend J. Richard Drees, superintendent of the Methodist Church Rock River Conference. Mrs. Blott remained as assistant director. In 1969, Mrs. Drees resigned to be married and Dorothy Blott, Wesley's perennial volunteer, became director of volunteers.

HEALING THE WHOLE PATIENT

A quiet but valued patient service was provided by Wesley's chaplain, Robert A. Dahl, who, for 20 years had given strength to frightened patients and wise advice to families, helping them to shoulder grief that seemed too much to bear. Chaplain Dahl recalled that he had averaged 45 visits a day with patients, their families and employees needing help. He estimated that he had made over 200,000 such calls, often bringing him to the hospital late at night. He said that the problems he most often dealt with were (1) discussing death with the patient who knew he was terminal, (2) helping the patient's family deal with the patient's illness, (3) helping married couples solve domestic problems and avert divorce, and (4) dissuading a patient from taking his own life. Wesley's beautiful chapel, which seated 50, was a tribute to Chaplain Dahl and the Woman's Auxiliary, whose hard work brought in the major part of the $40,000 necessary to build it in 1959. The first chapel had been a 9 by 12-foot office-chapel.

On Sunday morning the Reverend Dahl preached to a congregation of mostly wheelchair patients, brought to the chapel by high school students whom he had organized to serve as volunteers. There was joy in the chapel when nurses on the hospital staff, residents, interns or regular employees exchanged marriage vows. Some brought their babies back for Chaplain Dahl to baptize.

Chaplain Dahl was pleased with Wesley's ecumenical propensity. The pastors of at least ten denominations as well as priests and rabbis often came to visit patients. All were warmly welcomed at the Hospital. In 1968 Dahl extended an invitation to his colleagues to attend a get-acquainted meeting at Wesley. This was the first of a series of in-service sessions to help clergymen keep abreast of interdisciplinary healing and curing techniques employed in the modern hospital. "Religion and Psychiatry" was the first topic. Nine chaplains and pastors who regularly visited patients at Wesley attended the first meeting, including: Dr. Jerome Kaufman, Lutheran Charities Federation, chaplain for Lutheran patients at Wesley and Passavant hospitals; Rev. Herman Seinwerth, Chicago Temple; Rev. James Penn, St. James Cathedral; Rev. Glenn S. Sutton, Broadway Methodist; Father Eugene Durkin, Holy Name Cathedral; Rev. Donald Everhart, Protestant chaplain, Veterans Administration Hospital; Rev. Raymond Tillrock, deacon, Holy Name Cathedral; Assistant Chaplain Ronald Dixon, and Chaplain Dahl, Wesley.

A NURSE OF GREAT INFLUENCE

Nurses at Wesley and throughout the country were grieved to learn of the death of Bertha L. Knapp Smith August 1, 1965, at the age of 85. She was superintendent of nursing and nursing education at Wesley from 1908 to 1943 when she retired and was given the title of superintendent of nursing, emeritus, for life. In 1958 she married her college sweetheart, Dr. Richard A. Smith, chief of survey for the Michigan State Geological Department, who predeceased her. She died in her home in Neillsville, Wisconsin.

Few women in the nursing field exercised wider influence, not only in Wesley but in the whole profession. Mrs. Smith had been assistant superintendent of nursing at University Hospital, Ann Arbor, Michigan, and a supervisor of the Chicago Visiting Nurse Association before joining Wesley. She was one of the first nurses appointed to the Board of Nurse Examiners of the State of Illinois under the Civil Administration Code.

In 1959 the Wesley Nurses Alumnae Association had commissioned the well-known artist, John Doctoroff, to paint a portrait in oils of Bertha L. Knapp Smith. The excellent likeness was unveiled by the artist himself at a Wesley alumnae banquet and later the painting was placed in the east corridor near the Nursing Office.

Toward the Future Chapter 22

Wesley's participation in the Northwestern University Medical Center had been approved in principle by its Board of Trutees in 1963 and had been effective in some areas. Informal cooperation between the five affiliated institutions—Chicago Wesley Memorial Hospital, Children's Memorial Hospital, Evanston Hospital, Northwestern University and Passavant Memorial Hospital—resulted in substantial reductions in cost of x-ray film, labor-saving disposable items and other supplies as well as in insurance.

Committees were examining duplication of services, the most critical being obstetrics and gynecology. Both Wesley and Passavant had maternity floors and the possibility of their consolidation had been considered in the past. In 1965 the university invited Wesley to join the Chicago Maternity Center and Passavant in a feasibility study of one facility to accommodate the three units on a site immediately east of Passavant and to share the expense thereof. Medical School Dean Richard H. Young reminded his fellow trustees at Wesley that "the University and Hospital are intertwined, partly by reason of the Deering Deed of Gift, also by the desire of the Wesley staff for teaching and research opportunities afforded by the medical school and by the university's desire to use Wesley's clinical facilities."

Many questions were raised as to the impact on Wesley, and the Hospital's responsibility to the community, to the medical school and to further development and improvement in patient care. Following prolonged conjecture, Wesley President William H. Alexander announced that "the present position is that Wesley will participate in the creation of a proposed medical center organization, but will retain its autonomy."

Speaking administratively, Superintendent Kenath Hartman pointed out that the combined obstetrical service would offer new advantages to the Hospital's teaching program, offer better patient service and free space for other uses at Wesley.

It was resolved that Wesley would participate in a study by Holabird and Root as to the architectural feasibility of a combined maternity center.

New Trustees Elected

Earl M. Schwemm, agency manager of the Chicago office of the Great West Life Assurance Co., and *Peter H. Merlin*, member of the law firm of Gardner, Carton, Douglas, Chilgren and Waud, were elected trustees at the annual meeting in Janaury, 1964. Mr. Merlin, who came to the United States from the Principality of Liechtenstein in 1950, was a graduate of the University of Geneva and the University of Michigan. His wife was the daughter of T. Philip Swift, also trustee. A third trustee, *Bishop Thomas M. Pryor*, head of the Chicago area Methodist Church and trustee of the Rock River Conference of the Methodist Church, was elected at a special meeting in October.

James S. Kemper, Jr., president of Lumberman's Mutual Casualty Company, was elected a trustee in 1965. He held an LL.B. degree from Harvard University and had practiced law in New York, Los Angeles and Chicago. He had shown much interest in local and national health as a director of the National Society for the Prevention of Blindness, the National Council on Alcoholism, the Rehabilitation Institute of Chicago and the Salvation Army. Kemper was a second generation trustee. His father, James Scott Kemper, Sr., U.S. Ambassador to Brazil, 1953-56, had joined the Wesley board in 1939 and had become a life member of the Wesley governing board in 1963.

Dr. Corliss D. Anderson, professor of finance at Northwestern University School of Business and past president of Investment Analysts of Chicago, was named to the board in 1966. He was a co-founder and for 11 years partner of Duff, Anderson and Clark, specialists in industrial securities.

Edward F. Swift, III, executive vice president of Swift & Company, was elected to the board at its annual meeting, January, 1967. A native Chicagoan, he had joined the Chicago plant of the meat packing firm in 1948 and had become manager of the Evansville, Indiana plant in 1955. He returned to Chicago and was elected assistant vice president in 1958 and executive vice president in 1964.

Swift was a graduate of Yale University and served overseas during World War II, attaining the rank of captain in the field artillery. He joined a long line of forebears who had been Wesley trustees, from his great grandfather Gustavus F. Swift who was elected in 1896, to his father, T. Philip Swift, 1954.

Two trustees elected in April, 1968, were *Melville H. Ireland*, president of the Truax-Traer Coal Company, a division of Consolidated Coal Company, and *Jack Brickhouse*, manager of sports, WGN, a Chicago radio and television announcer since 1940. Well-known in sports and entertainment, Brickhouse had been the genial master of ceremonies at several events benefiting Wesley.

Bylaws Amended for Staff Flexibility

Following the maternity center discussions, a significant step toward future co-operation was taken by the medical staff and announced by Chief of Staff Clinton L. Compere: The bylaws of the Wesley Medical Staff were amended to permit a staff member also to be on the regular active staff of another affiliated hospital in the Northwestern University group.

New Department Chairmen

Dr. John M. Beal, chairman of the department of surgery at Northwestern and chief of the department at Passavant since 1963, was appointed chairman of the surgery department at Wesley in 1964. Dr. Beal had received his B.S. and M.D. degrees from the University of Chicago. He was an intern at New York Hospital and remained on its surgical staff until returning to Chicago, except for four years in California on the staffs of Wadsworth General (Los Angeles) and St. John's Hospital (Santa Monica). *Dr. David N. Danforth*, chairman of the obstetrics and gynecology department at Evanston Hospital, a Northwestern affiliate, was appointed chairman of the same department at Wesley September 1, 1965. He succeeded

Dr. George H. Gardner, chairman since 1946, who had reached the mandatory age for retirement stipulated by the medical staff bylaws.

Dr. Danforth, grandson of Wesley's founder, Dr. Isaac N. Danforth, was born in Evanston and graduated from Northwestern with an M.D. degree and a Ph.D. degree in physiology. He interned at New York Post-Graduate Hospital and was a resident physician at Sloane Hospital for Women, Columbia University. In World War II, Dr. Danforth served in the U.S. Navy. Upon his return he began practice at Wesley with Dr. Gardner, transferring to Evanston the following year. In 1966, he was elected a director of the American Board of Obstetrics and Gynecology. He was editor of *Textbook of Obstetrics and Gynecology* published by Harper & Row, containing contributions of 43 leading teachers and clinicians representing 30 teaching institutions.[1]

Dr. Guy F. Hollifield, medical director at the University of Virginia Hospital since 1955, was named chairman of Wesley's department of medicine July 1, 1966, succeeding Dr. Paul S. Rhoads, who had reached the age of retirement according to the staff bylaws. Dr. Hollifield received his M.D. degree from the University of Virginia in 1950, interned at Minneapolis General Hospital and was a fellow in internal medicine at the hospitals of the Universities of Minnesota and Virginia 1951-1954.

Dr. Rhoads had arrived at Wesley December 6, 1941, the day before the building was occupied. He was named chairman of medicine in 1943 and was chief of staff in 1945 and 1946. As retiring chairman of medicine, he received a $25,000 grant from the Standard Oil (Indiana) Foundation to expand Wesley's physicians' library and the medical records library.

Dr. James E. Eckenhoff, named chairman of anesthesia at Northwestern and chief of the division at Passavant, January, 1965, also became chairman of Wesley's anesthesia department the following year, replacing Dr. Mary Karp who had resigned. Dr. Karp had joined Wesley's staff in 1935 and had been anesthesia chairman since 1942. Dr. Eckenhoff was a 1941 graduate of the University of Pennsylvania School of Medicine, was a fellow of the Royal College of Surgeons which awarded him the Hunterian Professorship. He later served as clinical assistant in anesthesia at Queen Victoria Hospital in England.

---

[1] *The textbook was in its fourth edition when this book went to press.*

Coronaries Strike Two in Two Days

Heart attacks claimed the lives of two attending staff physicians within two days in 1965. On March 26 Dr. Gilbert H. Marquardt, medicine, was stricken in his home and died the same day; on March 27 *Dr. Robert T. McElvenny*, orthopedics, died of a heart attack at Wesley.

Dr. Marquardt, who joined Wesley in 1932, was chief of staff 1941-1942 and 1946-1947. A Northwestern graduate, he held the Elizabeth J. Ward Fellowship in medicine at the school from 1929 to 1932. In World War II he was a lieutenant colonel and chief of the army air force medical department, and in the Korean conflict he was a medical advisor to the air force surgeon general.

Dr. McElvenny joined Wesley's staff in 1941. He specialized in hip and spine surgery and was credited with pioneering in the field. He was a graduate of the University of Colorado Medical School and a diplomate of the American Board of Orthopedic Surgery.

Heart Station Director Named

Dr. Sheldon H. Steiner, former director of the cardiovascular research registry at the University of Indiana Heart Research Center, was appointed director of the Wesley Heart Station in 1966. A graduate of New York University, he had interned at Duke University Hospital and was a post-doctoral cardiopulmonary research trainee at the University of Indiana. From 1958 to 1960 he was research internist at the Wright Air Development Center, Dayton, Ohio, where he helped select the original crew of Mercury astronauts. He studied the effects of acceleration and gravity on the heart and circulation and personally submitted to 17 g's of force.

New Suite for Neurosurgery

The neurosurgical operating suite, long the dream of Dr. Paul C. Bucy, chief of Wesley's neurosurgical section, Dr. Daniel Ruge and other neurosurgeons on the medical staff, was dedicated January 17, 1966. Dr. Bronson Sands Ray, director of the neurosurgery department at New York Hospital—Cornell Medical Center since 1948 and a world leader in his specialty, was the speaker. Dr. Ray, who interned at Wesley (1928-1929) and had residencies at Passavant and Peter Bent Brigham (1929-1935), lauded Wesley's foresight in providing the facility. He told of the important role Northwestern and Wesley neurosurgeons and researchers had played in advancing knowledge in spinal cord and brain surgery.

Ninety guests inspected the unit, which consisted of two operating rooms plus control, utility, anesthesia and scrub rooms. The larger room and control center were sheathed in sheet steel to prevent interference from outside the room which could cause malfunction in neurosurgical electronic equipment.

Both operating and anesthesia rooms had overhead tracks from which hung movable and adjustable supports for intravenous fluids and other equipment. The tracks were first developed at Wesley to enable neurosurgeons to take advantage of recent surgical advances.

The smaller operating room was equipped to treat such conditions as Parkinson's disease, epilepsy and mental disease. An image intensifier, suspended from a ceiling track, revolved 360 degrees. The $25,000 intensifier was a gift from the Colonel Robert R. McCormick Charitable Trust of the Chicago Tribune Company. The Ode D. Jennings Trust gave $50,000 toward the total of $190,000 and the remainder was provided by the Wesley Service League and numerous individuals.

MEDICARE ARRIVES

Medicare slipped silently through Wesley's front door at nine a.m., July 1, 1966; past television cameramen, news photographers and reporters waiting for the crowds. However, no senior citizen waited to seize advantage of this socio-political phenomenon. The advent of Medicare was as unobtrusive at Wesley as it was at Passavant across the street and thousands of hospitals across the country.

A panel of Wesley trustees, administrators, medical staff members and nurses met in October to discuss experiences and observations during the first four months of Medicare. Participants were William H. Alexander, president of the Board of Trustees, Stuart S. Bell, chairman of the trustee nursing committee; Clay E. Steele, chairman of the trustee budget sub-committee; Kenath Hartman, hospital superintendent; Harold J. Straidl, comptroller; Dr. James B. Hurd, chief of staff; Dr. John M. Beal, chairman, department of surgery; Dr. Guy Hollifield, chairman, department of medicine; Dr. Jacob R. Suker, coordinator of medical training programs; and Mrs. Vera Thompson, director of nursing. Portions of their comments reveal Wesley's acceptance of the new plan to assure the well-being of a generation of people.

Mr. Alexander: Medicare, one of the significant innovations of our generation, came in quietly. But in the background a big job of preparation by hospital, medical, governmental, and health insurance personnel had been done.

Dr. Hurd: It was obvious to us that July 1 would not bring a fresh flow of patients. First, nobody likes to go to the hospital three days before a major holiday. Second, Wesley has been pressed to capacity for several years; 90 percent of our beds were occupied. It should be stressed that the Medicare patient receives the same fine care as any other patient. Over the years this also has been true of patients in charity and teaching beds.

Mr. Steele: Our figures reveal how vast the program must be nationally. During the first four months, Wesley cared for 1,530 Medicare patients. The total bills amounted to $985,133; the total collected was $706,186. The average stay was 17.2 days; the average cost was $644. We get some idea of the magnitude of Medicare when we consider that about 19,000,000 people are 65 years or older.

Mr. Staidl: Mr. Steele mentioned Medicare billing. In August we became hard-pressed financially. Payment from the government was less than half our billing. To meet salaries and other expenses we were forced to borrow $200,000 in short term loans in a tight money market. These loans have now all been paid.

Dr. Beal: We now have more long-stay patients, 30 days or more, than ever before. This October we had 114 long-stay cases. During the 12 months before Medicare, the average was 90 cases a month. This causes the long wait prior to admitting. A year ago, it was 10 days; now it is 22.

Dr. Hollifield: Speaking of long stays, our utilization committee is studying these cases and bringing action to bear where Medicare requirements are not met. The committee monitors admissions, discharges, emergencies and long-stay cases. The latter require attending physician certification and committee concurrence before the government will pay. The committee consists of 14 medical staff members and representatives of admitting, nursing, medical records, and administration.

Dr. Suker: What effect does Medicare have on the resident-intern program? At Wesley we have no ill effects. Full Medicare responsibilities have been accepted by the attending staff; the house staff continues to be responsible for care of patients without respect to classification.

Mrs. Thompson: In nursing at Wesley, as at every hospital in America, we could do with more help, particularly registered and licensed practical nurses. We established a coordinator pilot program on the sixth floor. A coordinator is responsible for all non-nursing activities, including admission, transfer, discharge of patients, physical environment, supply inventory, and supervision of station clerks and maids. Nurses are thus relieved to devote their time to patient care. The program is being expanded.

Mr. Bell: The trustees' nursing committee made a survey of where we get nurses, where we use them, and who they are. They are relatively young, single and mobile. For instance, 35 percent of our staff are graduates of the Wesley School of Nursing, 56 percent were employed immediately upon graduation; 20 percent have over 5 years of experience before coming to Wesley. The average age of our present staff is 27, and 87 percent are single. Relocation outside of Chicago was the most common reason for separation—27 percent for that reason. Marriage accounted for 15 percent of the terminations.

Mr. Hartman: Admittedly, there are problems—problems of obsolete equipment, personnel shortages, and difficulties in financing. This past year many of the professional and administrative staffs were interviewed by consulting architects to ascertain needs for the years ahead. Their requests are far-reaching in scope, size and cost.

THE CHANGING NEIGHBORHOOD
The community Wesley served, based on Federal Census reports, was called the Near North Side area and was bounded by the Chicago River on the south, the river's north branch on the west, North Avenue and Lake Michigan. When Wesley dedicated its 23-story Bedford stone building in 1941, it stood tall with Northwestern University, the Tribune Tower, the Wrigley Building, Furniture Mart and Palmolive Building. In later years Wesley was dwarfed by such giants as the Marina Towers, the Continental Plaza Hotel, and the 100-story John Hancock center, together housing thousands of new high-rise dwellers—Wesley's new neighbors and potential patients.

In an area 12 blocks long and 11 blocks wide, commercial and institutional construction permits were let totaling approximately $1.3 billion in the eleven years between January 1, 1957 and December 31, 1968, according to the Chicago Real Estate Board. Wesley and other institutions on the Northwestern campus contributed to the building boom: Wesley with its $7 million Allison Pavilion (1959), doctors' offices and patient rooms; Passavant with its $4 million Russell Tyson Pavilion (1958), expanded patient services and teaching units, and the $4½ million Ode D. Jennings Pavilion, doctors' offices and patient rooms (1966); and Northwestern with its Searle building (1965) for multiple medical school needs, all added to Chicago's jagged skyline.

One block north of Wesley and two blocks east to Lake Shore Drive, adjacent to the Chicago landmark, the Lake Shore Club,[1] was the 12-story American Hospital Association headquarters building (1958) and 10-story addition (1969) contiguous to its main building and adjacent to the Passavant nurses' residence. Both AHA buildings had two-story garages below ground level.

Wesley had purchased the 18-story Hampshire House at 201 East Delaware as a residence for student nurses and the 180 East Delaware building next to the Continental Plaza Hotel to house married residents and their families. It also owned three graystone buildings, circa 1900, adjacent to the Hospital at 226-228-230 East Superior Street which were used for supplemental living quarters for house staff and registered nurses and for additional research laboratories. In 1963, the Hospital bought the Gideons International Building at 212 East Superior Street for $270,000 and in 1965 had acquired the 7-story American Dental Association building at 222 East Superior Street at a cost of $1 million. The handsome building added 75 feet of frontage to the 80 feet already owned by Wesley.

The 222 Building, as it was known, relieved some of the pressure from the bulging main building. A second-story heated bridge connected the two structures, serving as a means of transport for patients, employees, pneumatic tubes, transcription lines, telephone and electric wires. The attractive first floor reception center became personnel offices, briefing rooms and a computer center. The second and part of the fifth floors contained 75 percent of student nurses' classroom activity and the third floor housed automated medical records and the doctors' library. Offices for

[1]*Northwestern University purchased the Lake Shore Club in 1978.*

doctors and management services were on the fifth and sixth floors along with two diagnostic laboratories and classrooms. The bridge and remodeling cost $120,000. The Hospital board had an eye on the 26-story Carriage House and made an offer in 1963, but negotiations failed in April, 1964, and the matter was considered closed at that time.

Expanding and Updating   Chapter 23

Wesley's Cathedral of Healing, a center of modernity in 1941, was inadequate for patient needs 25 years later. To repair the gap and make long-range plans, trustees named a Development Committee in 1966 chaired by T. Stanton Armour. The first step was to employ the firm, Walter Darling and Associates, to define the needs and arrange the mechanics of a fund-raising campaign. The hospital industrial engineers and planners, E. Tod Wheeler, associated with Perkins and Will, architects, were added to the Darling staff to create a program from the recommendations of the medical and administrative staffs, as well as the board of trustees.

While studies were under way, the trustees voted to update several areas in the main building vital to the Hospital's operation. Work began immediately on the following projects, some of which would take two to three years to complete:

Automated Elevators—Conversion of the five central core elevators to permit an efficiency gain of 20 percent in the grossly inadequate system. The change-over would take six months per elevator. Total cost—$215,000.

New Laundry—After studying and rejecting contractual laundry services, trustees voted to modernize its obsolete equipment. Cost—$220,000.

Telephone Service—Direct dialing for patients and additional terminals throughout the Hospital to facilitate communications. Cost—$3,000.

Complete Tuckpointing—For the first time in the building's 26 years of existence, the entire exterior was to be tuckpointed at one time. Cost—$17,000.

New Furniture—For patient comfort and aesthetics, the 1,016 items of matching furniture placed in all patient rooms provided the best improvement. All rooms were completely redecorated. Cost—$155,000.

Computer System—An IBM 360-30 computer was on order to replace a 1401 computer installed in 1964 and already running at capacity. Rental—$108,000 annually.

The Question of Costs

Part of the expenditure was met by gifts, part by operating income and a loan. Major donors for the immediate work were the Bazley Trust, $150,000 annually for 10 years to Wesley and Northwestern; William M. Allison endowment of $690,266; and Clara Nelson, who willed $143,232 for research.

The planners of Wesley's future were becoming increasingly concerned about rising costs for patients. At the close of the 1967 fiscal year, the average Wesley patient was paying a daily bed cost of $60. About $44 of this went for nursing, housekeeping and food costs. The remaining $16 was for such medical costs as laboratory, x-ray and medications. In a late summer survey, the Chicago Hospital Council revealed that Wesley's $60 per day stood below the median for Chicago. It was obvious, however, that the sophisticated electronic machines for modern medical methods, as well as for administrative work such as billing, could send costs out of sight. Moreover, technological change was so rapid that machines became obsolete in a short time.

Leasing was the Answer

Wesley found that it could rent machines and the owner would make repairs, replace parts and guarantee function. By 1968 Wesley had six pieces of expensive electronic equipment worth half a million dollars, with no investment, leased for a minimum of five years. Harold Staidl, comptroller, explained the advantages: "First, we recover our money quicker under lease cost than by depreciation; second, our medical staff works with the newest equipment available; third, conversion to new biomedical technology is more rapid when the owner, who usually is the manufacturer, does the converting; fourth, repair and replacement of parts is faster when the lessor is responsible."

At Wesley where 82 percent of patient bills were payable from third parties—Blue Cross/Blue Shield, private insurance, welfare agencies or Medicare—all billing was done by automated data processing. The detailed information required by third party payors was much more voluminous than the simple invoices of the past. It was estimated that 50 people would be required to get out the third party billing alone. With the rented IBM 360-30 computer ($108,000 annually) 25 persons did all the billing and other data processing. Wesley was the first hospital in Illinois to do all of its Medicare billing by computer.

The leasing policy opened new vistas at Wesley. In the radiology department, the 17-year-old fluoroscopic units on which radiologists turned out most of the 74,000 diagnostic x-rays in 1967, at a sacrifice of time and image sharpness, were replaced with *new fluoroscopic machines* on lease. Even more exciting was a newly developed *polytomograph* for body section radiology, which had been rented without the need for immediate cash.

A boon to cancer patients in the radiation therapy center was the 80-treatment-a-day *linear accelerator* which soon would double the 17,000 radiation treatments given the previous year. Waiting rooms and space for the new therapeutic machine were doubled at a cost of $250,000, but the expensive device itself was rented. The accelerator replaced the cobalt unit purchased in 1958. In explaining the difference, Dr. William T. Moss, chairman of the department of therapeutic radiology, said that cobalt (gamma) source of power begins to decrease with use, while the accelerator source remains constant and the rays more evenly distributed.

In the pathology department the new *12-channel auto-analyzer* was producing from one blood sample 12 different tests simultaneously for $12 to the patient, instead of the former four different blood tests ($3.50 each) for $14. Twelve tests individually would have cost $42 with the old method. The analyzer's value was further enhanced by hooking it with an *IBM 1080 computer* which would store and immediately retrieve data related to each patient's blood tests, offering many statistical advantages.

Another sophisticated newcomer to pathology was the *EM 300 electron microscope* which was equally valuable in diagnosing disease and in teaching.

Both the IBM 1080 computer and the EM 300 electron microscope were obtained on rental contracts.

MAJOR IMPROVEMENTS MADE

A new *cardiovascular laboratory* scheduled for completion in 1969 at a cost of $300,000 was expected to triple the work done in the old one built in 1959 for $56,000. Heart deficiencies to be studied and diagnosed included (1) valvular diseases, the most commonly known being rheumatic fever, (2) coronary arterial disease, or hardening of the arteries, (3) lesions in the cardiac muscle, (4) congenital heart disease in adults and children, the most frequent being the blue baby. It was said that the new unit would enable heart specialists to complete catheterization, any cine-coronary angiography procedure for most types of clinical heart disease then known. The average of 100 open heart surgeries performed annually at Wesley was expected to increase. When the new laboratory opened, the old heart station became a backup facility.

A new unit to measure pulmonary function, the *Esther Evans Emphysema Laboratory*, promised new hope for patients with respiratory problems. The patient breathed into a respirometer next to a table-top computer into which was fed the measurements of his lung capacity and condition. The machine instantaneously computed the data and recorded it on a card which was placed in the patient's chart. The procedure formerly took the physician an hour or more. The laboratory was the gift of friends of the national golf champion, Charles "Chick" Evans, whose wife, Esther, died of emphysema at Wesley in 1966. Personal appeal letters from Evans to hundreds of his friends in the sports world brought in funds for respirometers, treadmills and other devices with which to diagnose the hated pulmonary disease.

WESLEY MADE NO LITTLE PLANS

While the aforementioned improvements were under way, the trustee development committee and consultants were preparing to exceed all past Wesley achievements, incorporating advances and coordinating them with all member institutions of the Northwestern University Medical Center. One by one the planners, under the direction of T. Stanton Armour, committee chairman, consulted 150 members of Wesley's 17 medical departments and sections to learn their needs and how best to meet them. They exhaustively studied the issues of air rights over streets and alleyways and zoning which had to be changed in some areas. To preclude possible threats to completion, trustee Henry E. Seyfarth assigned the services of Joseph E. Wyse, specialist in zoning regulations and member of the firm of Seyfarth, Shaw, Fairweather and Geraldson, to the massive project. The planners obtained the endorsement of the Hospital Planning Council of Metropolitan Chicago and explored sources of funding, from federal government agencies to commercial, industrial and individual donors. Recent land acquisitions to the west along Superior Street gave Wesley slightly more than the 2.2 acres of land necessary to qualify for "Area Developments" and the right to negotiate or comply with the special regulations for overall land usage.

BOARD PROJECTS TEN-YEAR PROGRAM

A $31 million expansion and renewal plan for Chicago Wesley Memorial Hospital was announced January 24, 1969, by William H. Alexander, president of the Board of Trustees. The ten-year program called for modernizing existing buildings and expanding patient accommodations, changing the 700-bed hospital to an ultramodern 1,000-bed institution.

The first phase in the long-range plan would be accomplished in three steps westward from the main building. Step one was an 18-floor tower making 300 additional beds available. Step two was razing the three remaining stone structures on Superior Street and building a second tower during the 1980s. Step three was remodeling the main building which had already begun.

There would be some changes in these ambitious plans but the razing of the stone buildings was partly accomplished almost immediately. Demolition began September 2 on the brownstones at 226, 228 and 230 Superior Street which had stood for decades, some said, "like warts on the hands of beautiful Wesley." They were destroyed in 10 days and converted into a temporary parking lot.

DR. EGEBERG'S OPTIMISTIC SEND-OFF

The capital campaign received a rousing kick-off at a dinner in the Grand Ballroom of the Drake Hotel September 24, 1969, attended by some 300

Wesley doctors, trustees, administrators, their spouses and guests. Dr. Roger O. Egeberg, assistant secretary for Health, Education and Welfare, Washington, D.C., honored his alma mater as guest speaker at the prestigious event. Board President Alexander was toastmaster and T. Stanton Armour outlined the fund raising plans. Medical staff spokesmen were Dr. Daniel Ruge[1], chief of staff, and Dr. Vincent J. O'Conor, Jr., chairman of the staff's development committee. Former congresswoman and trustee, Marguerite Stitt Church, spoke briefly with eloquent charm, and Trustee James S. Kemper, Jr., introduced Dr. Egeberg. Special guests were James G. Brawley, Chicago regional director of Health, Education and Welfare, and Hiram Sibley, executive director of the Hospital Planning Council of Metropolitan Chicago.

"Hospitals like Wesley are the backbone of patient care in this country," Dr. Egeberg informed his audience. "We look, not to D.C., but out where practice is being carried on. Wesley, as part of a great medical center, is a very important place to evolve new health care delivery. We can't produce many more doctors fast. The doctor's hands must be extended and he must be willing to have them extended by new care methods.

"That recognition and the national resolve to reach the goal of health care for all people is, to me, the most exciting and most challenging quest that medicine has ever begun. I will gladly accept the indictment of being an optimist because I think medicine will make it," Dr. Egeberg said.

Dr. Egeberg received his M.D. degree from Northwestern and interned at Old Wesley and New Passavant in 1929 and 1930. He was well remembered by nurse administrators, Emma Grimm and Coralie Bennett, who had recently celebrated their 35th anniversary as Wesley nurses. Miss Bennett said that the handsome six-foot-four Swede with a shy sense of humor had signed his name "Olaf" in her nursing school annual.

[1]*As White House physician, Dr. Daniel Ruge, neurosurgeon, guided the treatment of President Reagan's gunshot wound at The George Washington University Medical Center after the assassination attempt March 30, 1981. His insistence on adherence to routine was a major reason for the remarkable success. New York Times, April 11, 1981, by William A. Knaus, M.D. (Dr. Knaus was co-director of the intensive-care unit at The George Washington University Medical Center).*

"Dr. Ruge had been chosen White House physician because of his association with Dr. Loyal Davis, Nancy Reagan's father," Hugh Sidey, Time Magazine, April 13, 1981.

NUMC Efforts Reap Rewards   Chapter 24

As the largest clinical component of the Northwestern University Medical Center, Wesley's role in the center was its primary concern in charting its complicated course of expansion. Northwestern had organized the center as a separate legal entity in 1966 together with seven institutions which had affiliated with the university during the previous 66 years: Chicago Wesley Memorial Hospital, 1899; Passavant Memorial Hospital, 1925; Children's Memorial Hospital, 1946; Evanston Hospital, 1950; Veterans Administration Research Hospital, 1950; the Rehabilitation Institute of Chicago, 1960; and the Chicago Maternity Center (nucleus of Prentice Women's Hospital and Maternity Center)[1], 1966.

The purpose of the center was "to foster joint effort to provide centralized facilities and to improve teaching, research and patient care within the existing framework of private medicine and independently operated institutions."

Proposals to implement the aims were drafted in 1967. These included new structures for the Rehabilitation Institute and the aforementioned Women's Hospital and Maternity Center with a Psychiatric Institute also in the latter building. The university donated the land east of Passavant for the

---

[1]*Named for the hospital's generous benefactors, Mr. and Mrs. (Abbie) Rockefeller Prentice, whose deaths occurred four months apart in 1972. The Prentice Women's Hospital and Maternity Center was dedicated January 22, 1976.*

two new buildings. In 1968, the planning committee suggested that the city parking garage at the southwest corner of Fairbanks Court and Superior Street be acquired for the site of outpatient clinics. Dr. J. Roscoe Miller, chancellor of Northwestern University, was informed that the garage might be sold for a highrise apartment building, so he obtained trustee approval to purchase the eastern two-thirds of the parking site. At this point, Dr. Miller went directly to Mayor Richard J. Daley of Chicago and proposed that the city sell the garage to Northwestern. Dr. Miller emphasized that a new facility would provide health care for a heavily populated section of Chicago. Mayor Daley agreed and said that negotiations would be favorable.

THE McGAW MEDICAL CENTER OF NORTHWESTERN UNIVERSITY

One Northwestern trustee, who heard Chancellor Miller describe the potential of the Northwestern University Medical Center, was inspired to immediate and electrifying action. The trustee was Foster G. McGaw, who gave $10 million to ensure that the fervent desire of his long-time friend, "Rocky" Miller, could proceed on its way to realization. The gift from Mr. and Mrs. McGaw was designated for "health center planning." Intended for joint programming and centralization of services among the eight member institutions, the funds were not to be used for capital development. In appreciation, the center was named the Northwestern University—McGaw Medical Center.

McGaw, board chairman of the American Hospital Supply Corporation, said that he and his wife, Mary, hoped to see the health center emerge as a cooperative venture of great stature during their lifetime. Subsequently, the McGaws gave a second $10 million. At that time, the name of the center was changed to the McGaw Medical Center of Northwestern University.

Dr. Richard H. Young, dean of Northwestern University Medical School, had relinquished his position as director of the medical center in 1969 and was replaced by Ray E. Brown, who became vice president of the McGaw Medical Center. Brown, who had extensive experience in hospital administration at the University of Chicago, Duke University and the Affiliated Hospitals Center in Boston, supported Dr. Miller's personal commitment to the McGaw Medical Center and moved energetically to carry out the high-reaching plan.

Wesley and Unionization

The excitement of Wesley's bright expectations had been tempered by an ongoing labor dispute with HELP (Hospital Employees Labor Program) which reached climactic force in early 1970. Between 1967 and 1970, HELP had intermittently distributed pro-union flyers outside the Hospital, aimed at Wesley's 1500 employees.

On November 26, 1969, the same day that the Illinois Supreme Court handed down a decision giving South Chicago Community Hospital employees the right to strike, Wesley's superintendent, Kenath Hartman, received a letter from HELP's president urging the Hospital to accept HELP as the employee bargaining agent. The proposal was rejected on the grounds that no evidence existed that the majority of employees desired a union. In January the union claimed to have 800 cards from employees and, unless the hospital negotiated, a strike would be called. After several exchanges between the Hospital and the union, a strike was called and picket lines set up on February 5, 1970. Despite efforts to stop entry of supplies, Wesley functioned smoothly and patient care was not affected.

Picketing ceased on February 9 after Wesley appealed to the Circuit Court and agreed to hold an election jointly with the union. The election, held February 24-26, was said to be fraught with irregularities which Wesley protested.

Picketing and appeals continued until November 25, when the Circuit Court issued a restraining order limiting picketing to six persons per entrance and forbidding unlawful interference with staff, suppliers or vendors entering or exiting the hospital. All picketing was stopped December 15 and striking employees were reinstated, until the Appellate Court handed down a decision. Wesley appealed to the Illinois Supreme Court, but no action was taken until March 14, 1972, when members of HELP ratified a two-year contract with the Hospital. The contract, which covered approximately 700 nonprofessional employees at Wesley, would be in effect until January 14, 1974.

The Power of a Storm

The violence of the sixties was nowhere more evident than in the elements when the snowstorm of the century paralyzed Chicago, January 27-29, 1967. Thanks to the spirit of cooperation and sacrifice at Wesley, patient service was not curtailed, even at the blizzard's peak. Stranded employees shifted to the unfilled jobs of those who could not reach the Hospital. Student nurses were dismissed from classes to work on patient floors, capably filling a big gap in the nursing staff.

The dietary department had the greatest shortage, but some workers already on hand at the storm's start worked 24 hours straight. Many other departments filled in so that every patient received his regular three hot meals a day during the storm. About 50 employees slept in the lobby or on cots in the solarium. Comptroller Don Bloom did an eight-hour stretch as an orderly in the psychiatric department. The usually active admitting department was deserted. New patients could not get to the Hospital and discharged ones had no way to leave.

At nursing station 6 East, they found a million dollar worker from a Wisco Hardware store. Actually, John A. Fitschen, president and general manager of the Wisco Hardware Company, Madison, Wisconsin, one of the state's largest wholesale firms, was stranded in a nearby hotel during the 23-inch snowfall. He made his way to Wesley and said to Superintendent Hartman, "I'll be hanged if I'll sit in my room all day and watch TV. I heard on the radio that you need help. Put me to work." Within half an hour, the nurses on 6 East had a highly proficient station clerk. Mr. Fitschen worked steadily from 8 a.m. to 4:30 p.m. keeping records, carrying food trays, fulfilling patient needs and assisting nurses. He was one of many visitors who gladly subbed for snowbound employees that particular weekend in Wesley's history.

NEW TRUSTEES

Four business and professional men elected to the Wesley Board of Trustees at its annual meeting January 13, 1969, included the following: *Roy M. Fisher*, editor and vice president of the Chicago *Daily News*, a Harvard Neiman Fellow and lecturer at the Northwestern Medill School of Journalism; *Austin Fleming*, legal authority on trusts and federal taxation with the Northern Trust Company; *Roy H. Krueger*, vice president of Browne and Storch Realtors, president of the Board of Trustees of the Old People's Home; *Edgar Peske*, vice president and treasurer of Illinois Bell Telephone Co., a trustee of Roosevelt University and a director of the Hospital Planning Council of Metropolitan Chicago.

NEW APPOINTMENTS

Dr. George A. Sisson was appointed chairman of the Wesley department of otolaryngology September 18, 1968, after serving in the same capacity at the Community General Hospital in Syracuse, New York. He was a governor of the advisory committee of otolaryngology for the American College of Surgeons, a member of the board of examiners of the American Board of Otolaryngology, and on the advisory committee for communicative disorders at the National Institutes of Health.

Dr. Geoffrey Kent, an Englishman born in Holland and a naturalized American citizen since 1953, became director of Wesley's department of pathology in September, 1969. His English parents lived in Amsterdam, where he was born, reared and graduated from the University of Amsterdam Medical School. He served a residency in pathology at the Manchester Royal Infirmary, 1940-44, was in the Royal Army Medical Corps, 1944-1947, and was a resident in pathology at the London Hospital, 1947-1950. He moved to Chicago in 1953 and became associate director of pathology at Cook County Hospital until 1958, then was pathology director at West Suburban Hospital until his appointment at Wesley.

Dr. John J. Bergan was appointed director of the transplantation division at Northwestern University Medical Center which included work at Wesley, Passavant and Children's hospitals. He also was named director of the International Organ Transplant Registry of the American College of Surgeons-National Institutes of Health.

THREE GRANDSONS OF EARLY TRUSTEES SUCCUMB

The latter half of the decade brought the deaths of three highly esteemed Wesley trustees, George William Dixon, 58, on July 21, 1966, his cousin, Wesley Moon Dixon, 73, on November 3, 1969 and, just two weeks later, T. Philip Swift, 78, on November 17. The Dixons were grandsons of Arthur Dixon, founder of the Dixon Transfer Co., who joined the Wesley board in 1899 and served until his death in 1917. Philip Swift was the grandson of Gustavus F. Swift, founder of Swift & Co., who was a trustee from 1896 until he died in 1903.

Philip Swift was a director of Swift & Co., and vice president of Continental Illinois Bank & Trust Company. He was survived by his wife; two sons, Edward F. Swift III, who also was a Wesley trustee, and Phelps

Hoyt Swift; and a daughter, Mrs. Peter H. Merlin, whose husband was a trustee.

George Dixon, an attorney with degrees from Northwestern, was chairman of the Wesley board's budget committee when he died suddenly in his home in Winnetka. He was named to the executive committee in 1941 and from 1942 to 1951 was the board's vice president. His wife, Margaret, was a member of the service league and recently had been general chairman of its successful Tattoo benefit. His father and mother, George W. Dixon, Sr., and Marion M. Dixon, were presidents of the Wesley board of trustees and the Ladies Aid Society respectively. His sister, Mrs. (Marion) Stanley B. Zaring, had been elected a trustee in 1956.

Wesley Moon Dixon, graduate of Cornell University and president of Container Corporation of America since 1947, came on the Wesley Board in 1949. He also served as a director of Harris Trust and Savings Bank, Pure Oil Company and U.S. Gypsum. He was a life trustee of Northwestern University and had been president of the board from 1959 to 1964. He was the son of Thomas John and Dora (Moon) Dixon and in 1926 was married to Katherine S. Strawn, daughter of Silas Hardy Strawn. They had three sons, Wesley Moon, Steward Strawn and Thomas Hardy.

The elder son, Wesley Moon Dixon, Jr., was married to Suzanne Searle and it was she who carried on the family heritage of volunteer hospital service. She was elected to the Passavant Woman's Board in 1961 and worked on many committees, including serving as chairman of the Passavant Cotillion. In 1975, Mrs. Wesley M. Dixon, Jr. became president of the Northwestern Memorial Hospital[1] Woman's Board, formed by combining the Wesley Woman's Board and the Passavant Woman's Board, and was named a member of the new hospital's Board of Trustees.

In Memoriam

A. Newell Rumpf, President of Harris Trust and Savings Bank and treasurer of the Wesley board of trustees since 1962, died suddenly February 3, 1968, in New York City where he was attending a banking convention. He devoted much of his time to the Boy Scouts and the Chicago Urban League.

Charles O. Loucks, Chicago attorney for 65 years and Wesley trustee since

[1]*Northwestern Memorial Hospital was created in 1972 by the consolidation of Wesley Memorial and Passavant Memorial Hospitals.*

1942, died on Christmas Day, 1967, at the age of 90. For the past 25 years he had gratuitously handled legal aspects of all wills and bequests for the benefit of the Hospital, as well as its corporate tax problems.

Dr. Thomas C. Laipply, director of Wesley's pathology department and professor at Northwestern University, died of a heart attack February 3, 1967. He established Wesley's School of Medical Technology and was commissioner of continuing education for the American Society of Clinical . Pathology. He had published 58 papers on pathology subjects.

Guidelines to Greatness   Chapter 25

The Wesley Board of Trustees began the decade of 1970 by renovating its own bylaws and those of the Wesley Society, the Hospital's corporate body. It was said that more policy statements had been added, deleted or streamlined over the past year than at any time within memory. Committees of the medical staff also reviewed, renewed and revised their rules and regulations to meet requirements of medical advances and the growing number of patients.

Hospitals and the public were well aware of the universal medical evolution. The wide variety of services available to and demanded by individual patients, inner city participation in the health care system, government intervention through Medicare and other national health programs all created anxieties and increased tension for health care providers.

REORGANIZATION

Wesley coped with difficult problems by reorganizing on a corporate level to redistribute part of the load carried by the president of the Board of Trustees and the superintendent of the Hospital. At the top of administration, the trustees added a new position, a full time president and executive officer. The new president was *John C. Sturgis*, former vice president of the Continental Illinois National Bank and Trust Company of Chicago, whose appointment was effective September 1, 1970. Sturgis had been a trustee of Children's Memorial Hospital for 15 years and president for four years before coming to Wesley. He was vice president of the McGaw Medical Center of Northwestern University. *Kenath Hartman*, hospital superintendent since 1960 and assistant superintendent starting in 1948, was elected executive vice president responsible for daily operations.

The Board of Trustees increased its membership from 39 to 45 plus 14 life members. To give more flexibility in selecting trustee candidates qualified for greater community health participation, the new bylaws reduced the number of trustees required to be of the Methodist faith from two thirds to one half.

The bylaws called for three physicians, *the chief of staff, Dr. Melvyn A. Bayly; vice chief of staff, Dr. Jacques M. Smith;* and *chairman of the medical council, Dr. Guy Hollifield*, to be members of the board. As new officers were elected by the medical staff, they would replace the medical officers on the Board of Trustees.

The trustees completed the reorganization on a business corporate basis at the January 1971 annual meeting when *Edward F. Swift III*, executive vice president of Swift & Company, was elected chairman of the Wesley Board of Trustees. The new pattern had been established by outgoing president, William H. Alexander.

Five administrative officers were appointed vice presidents, and two were assistant vice presidents. The vice presidents were *Harold Staidl*, finance; *Donald Bloom*, administration; *John Wingerton*, plant operations, *Vera Thompson*, patient care and nursing education, and *Marlin Barklage*, personnel. The assistant vice presidents were *William Mumma* and *Russell Colling*, both in plant operations.

Ronald D. Olmsted, former associate director of development at the University of Chicago, was appointed vice president for development and public relations in July, 1971. Before moving from California to Chicago in 1968, he had been executive director of the Los Angeles Center for International Visitors for seven years.

New Trustees on Enlarged Board

The increased Board of Trustees provided places for six additional members and the death of one trustee left seven vacancies, an unusually large class of trustees. The following were elected in 1970: *William B. Browder*, vice president and general counsel of Trans Union Corporation, past president of the Chicago Crime Commission and the Mid-American chapter of the American Red Cross; *George E. Johnson*, president of the Johnson Products Company, cosmetic firm, president of the Independence Bank of Chicago, past president of the Urban League of Chicago, also one of nine persons nominated by President Nixon to serve on the board of governors of the United States Postal Service; *Frederick Liechty*, senior vice president for marketing of the Chicago Blue Cross Plan and former business manager of the University of Michigan Hospital, also board chairman of the United Methodist Church of Evanston; *James F. Oates, Jr.*, attorney, past board chairman and chief executive officer of the Equitable Life Assurance Society of the United States, past president of the Chicago Bar Association and the YMCA of Chicago, also a Northwestern graduate with honorary degrees from 11 universities and colleges; *Elroy C. Sandquist*, graduate of Northwestern law school and the U.S. Naval Academy, director of Hull House Association and the Welfare Council of Metropolitan Chicago, vice president of Lake Bluff and Chicago Homes for Children; *Paul M. Steinbrink*, vice president and treasurer of Swift & Company, trustee of the Methodist Old Peoples Home; *Gordon R. Worley*, vice president for finance of Montgomery Ward & Company and its subsidiary, Marcor, Inc., director of the Chicago Dental Hygiene Association and trustee of Garrett Theological Seminary.

Three trustees elected to the board at the 1971 annual meeting were: *Henry Gardner*. a vice president of Continental Illinois National Bank and Trust Company between 1948 and 1969, then president of the National Boulevard Bank, active in the American Cancer Society, Chicago Crime Commission and Metropolitan Crusade of Mercy; *Lee Phillip*, well-known radio and television personality, in private life Mrs. William Bell, whose three children were born at Wesley; *Dempsey J. Travis*, president and board chairman of Sivage Mortgage Corp. and of the Travis Realty Co., member of the Presidential Task Force on Urban Renewal, past president of the Chicago NAACP, director of Cosmopolitan Chamber of Commerce, author of numerous articles about finances and the black community, also of the book, *Don't Stop Me Now*.

Trustees who died in 1970 and 1971 were *Arthur Dole, Jr.*, former president of the Wesley Board of Trustees, *Albert C. Buehler, Lanning MacFarland, Henry F. Tenney* and *Rawleigh Warner*.

At the 1972 annual meeting, five trustees were elected to the Wesley Board. They included *Dr. Judith S. Bensinger*, Northwestern graduate with B.S. and M.D. degrees, physician in the Head Start Services program, clinical director of the Land of Lincoln Goodwill Industries in Springfield, and member of Illinois State Commission on Children; *John J. Crown*, partner in the law firm of Jenner & Block, vice president of Henry Crown and Company, graduate of Northwestern law school, who practiced in state and federal courts, both trial and appellate; *Margaret E. Robson*, president of The Canyon, Inc., a group of 400 young business people interested in development and leadership of Chicago, 1956 to 1960, whose husband, John E. Robson, was Undersecretary of Transportation from 1968 to 1970; *David E. Stahl*, comptroller and director of financial management for the City of Chicago, graduate of Miami University in Ohio, named one of Chicago's Ten Outstanding Young Men in 1968, and vice president of Chicago Council of Boy Scouts of America; and *Dr. Arthur DeBoer*, Northwestern medical school graduate, specialist in open heart and vascular surgery at Wesley, who had recently been elected vice chief of staff.

DOCTORS REVISE BYLAWS

The medical staff simplified the committee structure in its bylaws to facilitate action when urgent situations demanded it. The bylaws of both the trustees and the medical staff were restructured to mesh with those of the McGaw Medical Center of Northwestern University.

Chief of Staff Melvyn A. Bayly appointed Dr. Richard E. Blonsky, neurologist, as chairman of Wesley's committee of 11 attending staff members to study community health planning. For years Wesley doctors had examined and treated indigent patients from areas west of the Hospital who came to the Northwestern clinics. Some Wesley physicians currently were associated with Erie Neighborhood House, Olivet Medical Center and the Flannery Senior Citizens Apartments. They desired to participate more extensively in the inner city health program. The need had been emphasized in 1969 when a crisis at Cook County threatened to close its doors and all Chicago hospitals were asked to take the county patients and assign them to staff doctors. The Wesley staff agreed but the emergency did not materialize. This proved the need for a city-wide cooperative plan, and the new committee wanted Wesley to cooperate fully and effectively. The committee members were: Drs. Blonsky, neurology; Whitney Addington, medicine; Patricia Field, psychiatry; C. Larkin Flanagan, medicine; Allwyn H. Gatlin, obstetrics-gynecology; Jerome C. Goldstein, otolaryngology; Michael C. Govostis, surgery; Wilson H. Hartz, Jr., medicine; Robert D. Keagy, orthopedics; James W. Nicklas, pediatrics; and Frederick W. Preston, surgery.

WESLEY/PASSAVANT STAFFS EXCHANGE PRIVILEGES

A growing spirit of cooperation within the medical center was exemplified by the agreement of Wesley and Passavant doctors to exchange medical staff privileges. Reciprocal arrangements permitted Wesley doctors to admit patients to Passavant and Passavant doctors to admit patients to Wesley.

Wesley president John C. Sturgis predicted that "open staff privileges between Wesley and Passavant doctors will be a benchmark in the annals of Northwestern's McGaw Medical Center." He added that consent among doctors of both institutions was unanimous.

"Under this arrangement a Passavant doctor with a patient who needs catheterization and open heart surgery can admit that patient to Wesley," John M. Stagl, executive vice president of Passavant, explained. "By the same token, a Wesley doctor with a patient who has extensive kidney problems and who might need dialysis or a kidney transplant, can be admitted to Passavant.

"In recent years each hospital has cooperated in building strong specialties not offered by the other. This new exchange of privileges makes full use of these diverse specialties," continued Mr. Stagl. "This is an example of two institutions voluntarily taking the step toward conservation of medical resources, not only in nonduplication of costly equipment, but in the most efficient use of health manpower."

DR. ECKENHOFF NAMED DEAN

Dr. James E. Eckenhoff, chairman of anesthesia at Wesley and at Northwestern was appointed dean of Northwestern University Medical School in February, 1970. He succeeded Dr. Richard H. Young, who had been dean since 1949 and resigned because of illness. Dr. Young had served as director of the Northwestern University Medical Center since it was first established as a legal entity in 1963. He died September 1, 1970.

Since coming to Wesley and Northwestern, Dr. Eckenhoff had developed an outstanding anesthesia resident training program and an inhalation therapy department. He also had directed Northwestern's NIH-supported Anesthesia Research Center, one of five in the United States.

NEW DEPARTMENT CHAIRMEN

Dr. Edward A. Brunner succeeded Dr. Eckenhoff as chairman of the anesthesia departments at Northwestern and at Wesley, where he also directed respiratory therapy. He was a graduate of Hahnemann Medical College, Philadelphia, with an M.D. degree and a Ph.D. in pharmacology. He did postgraduate work in biochemical effects of anesthetics on brain metabolism and was medical chairman of the medical student preceptor committee of the American Society of Anesthesiologists.

Dr. John Boehm became chairman of Wesley's pediatrics department in 1971 replacing Dr. L. Martin Hardy, who resigned. Dr. Boehm also was assistant dean for student affairs and associate professor of pediatrics, obstetrics and gynecology at the medical school. A graduate of the University of Notre Dame and of Northwestern Medical School, Dr. Boehm served a two-year residency in pediatrics at Children's Memorial Hospital, a McGaw Medical Center affiliate, and two years as chief of pediatrics, U.S. Army Hospital in Frankfurt am Main, Germany.

Dr. Samuel Bluefarb, chairman of the dermatology department at Northwestern, was appointed to the same position at Wesley. He earned his medical degree at the University of Illinois Medical School, interned at Cook County Hospital and took his resident training in dermatology at Bellevue Hospital in New York.

Dr. William J. Kane, formerly professor of orthopedic surgery at the University of Minnesota, was appointed chairman of the same department at Wesley. He succeeded Dr. Edward L. Compere, who retired after 29 years on the Wesley staff. Dr. Kane also was named Ryerson professor and chairman of the orthopedic department at Northwestern. A graduate of Columbia University's College of Physicians and Surgeons, Dr. Kane subsequently was associated with the University of Minnesota Hospitals, where he was director of the resident training program.

A Remarkable Transaction

The largest and most glamorous purchase of Wesley's 82-year history was the 26-story Carriage House at 215 E. Chicago Avenue, with only a 16-foot alley separating it from the Hospital. The attractive hotel with 299 apartments would permit the nursing school and all subsidized rentals to be under one roof with its own 224-car garage. An outside inn with cafe service facing a large swimming pool on the sixth floor, and an elite restaurant on the first floor were among the features expected to attract student nurses, R.N.'s, interns and residents. Among other benefits were direct access between the Hospital and Carriage House via the sixth floor bridge, providing more security and less travel time for employees. Other advantages to Wesley were the elimination of costly rental subsidies to private owners, removal of the need to refurnish Hampshire House and centralization of maintenance people responsible for one housing unit instead of several. The five-story garage helped Wesley fulfill city garage zoning regulations and provided building expansion space above the garage.

Wesley's interest in the site had predated its acquisition by nearly 30 years. When the new building was opened in 1941, trustees discussed the value of the adjacent vacant lot, but immediate needs precluded planning for the future. In 1945, a five-story garage was built on the lot and was purchased by Jack Galter the following year. In 1961, Galter and his wife watched with pride the construction of their imposing Carriage House. Wesley made its first offer in 1963 and the deal was off and on for seven years, culminating with the closure April 1, 1970.

It certainly was a formidable transaction for a hospital. However, considering the expediency, the trustees were convinced that Wesley's ownership of the Carriage House was the only sensible solution to its space problems. Part of the $10 million purchase price was met by exchanging Hampshire House with the Galters, and by selling the apartment at 180 East Delaware to the Great Western Hotel chain, owners of the adjacent Continental Plaza Hotel. In 1971, the Galters turned over to Hubert Howard, Wesley trustee property chairman, $50,000, the first of a series of donations from the Galters to Wesley.

The Carriage House manager, Robert Sweeney, his secretary, Grace Miller, and assistant manager, Dorothea McCann and others who wished to remain became Wesley employees. Previously, Wesley had housed 500 nurses, student nurses and house staff families in its own buildings or nearby private apartments. In addition it rented 200 car spaces from outside facilities. The Carriage House gave Wesley 50 addtional apartments, more parking spaces and substantial room for nursing school classrooms, libraries, recreational area and storage space.

Men Enroll as Wesley Student Nurses

The Wesley School of Nursing opened the 1971-72 school year with 256 students including 96 freshmen, the largest enrollment in more than five years. A significant innovation was the registration of two male student nurses, the first in the school's 80-year history. The young men were Ken Wheeler, an air force veteran, and Gale Richard Herring from Metropolis, Illinois.

Guest speaker for the first assembly was Vernice Ferguson, R.N., chief of nursing service at Veterans Administration West Side Hospital, and assistant professor at the University of Illinois College of Nursing. Miss Ferguson was the 1970 recipient of the Mary Mahoney Award from the American Nurses Association for "efforts toward integration of the nursing profession." The award was named for Mary Mahoney, America's first black nurse. It stated that Miss Ferguson was "a black who made it in nursing and . . . worked hard to . . . break down prejudice while building understanding." Miss Ferguson told the students that they must care enough to lead in improving the quality of nursing care. "Today's students in nursing will play an important role in designing a health care system, participating in its delivery, and evaluating the outcome," she predicted.

Lois Ebinger, director of the school, gave three reasons for the enrollment increase of the Wesley school, then the largest in an Illinois private hospital: (1) Cost problems had forced several schools in the Chicago area to close; (2) The rising cost of college tuition made Wesley's three-year nursing diploma program attractive to economy-minded parents and students; and (3) Wesley offered superior accommodations at the Carriage House.

Three nursing school classrooms were casualties when the linear accelerator was installed in their space in the Wesley basement. Classes were transferred to two 20 by 40-foot mobile rooms on the Fairbanks Court lawn facing Northwestern. They were electrically heated, air conditioned, with ample chalk and tack boards, but did nothing aesthetically for Wesley's Gothic lines.

Baby Boom Boosts Women's Hospital

More babies were born at Wesley during August, 1970, than in any month since the Hospital opened in 1888. The total number was 227 and 12 expectant mothers were routed to Passavant when Wesley's maternity beds were filled. Chief of staff Melvyn Bayly, himself an obstetrician, and Erma Rupp, supervisor on the obstetrical floor, projected these reasons for the increase: The Wesley prenatal clinics were serving more patients than ever before; The Maternity Center had decreased its number of home deliveries in favor of hospital deliveries of which Wesley traditionally had been the recipient; Wesley, along with other Chicago hospitals, was helping to lighten the load of Cook County and Provident hospitals, which were beset with financial and administration problems. The increased deliveries continued into 1971 and 1972, a strong endorsement for the Women's Hospital and Maternity Center[1] still on the drawing boards at that time.

[1]*Ground was broken on the site immediately east of Passavant in the summer of 1972 for the Women's Hospital and Maternity Center. It was completed and dedicated January 22, 1976, as the Prentice Women's Hospital and Maternity Center.*

Putting it All Together   Chapter 26

Wesley's projected building and other long-range plans were held in abeyance and development consultants were terminated after John Sturgis became president, but all improvements in the main building continued at full speed. Patient comfort was assured through a $1.9 million electrical renewal program which would provide air conditioners on all surgical, patient, and intensive care floors, electric beds for all patients and compliance with city electric and safety codes.

A trustee task force titled "Safeguarding Wesley Resources" was led by Melville H. Ireland, to retire a $3.5 million debt on the two buildings vital to daily operations, the Doctors Tower in the Allison Pavilion and the Carriage House.

PROBLEMS OF PRICE-WAGE FREEZE

A general salary increase in the winter of 1969 and a slump in the general labor market the following summer resulted in unusual employment stabilization. Job turnover was only half that of the late 1960s. This condition plus the Presidential price-wage freeze of August, 1971, forced Wesley to cut 12 percent from the employee budget. In order to meet the binding contract for renovation, it was necessary to terminate 213 full and part-time employees, with regrets. Patient care continued at a high level due to increased efforts and efficiency of the remaining personnel.

Day Surgery

Wesley initiated "day surgery" in November, 1971, whereby certain operations under general anesthesia were performed and the patients discharged in less than one day's time. Formerly patients were admitted in the afternoon prior to surgery and discharged at noon the day after surgery, requiring almost two full days and a night in the Hospital. Under the new system preoperative examinations were completed on an outpatient basis with major insurance companies altering their policies accordingly.

Advantages to the patient were smaller hospital bills, less time lost and fewer family disruptions. As for the Hospital, evening and night nurses were free for seriously ill patients, bed usage was improved since each bed could accommodate five surgical patients weekly instead of two or three, and housekeeping was simplified because rooms were prepared in the evening for use the next day. Procedures approved for day surgery were dilation and curettage (D&C), cysto and retrograde pyelography, excisions of benign and malignant skin lesions, minor orthopedic surgery, and minor hand and foot surgery.

Computerized Phones Due Soon

Wesley received welcome news in June that it would soon join Children's, Evanston and Passavant hospitals and Northwestern University in a computerized telephone switching system called Centrex I. The system included central paging accessible by telephone anywhere in the medical center. The names and telephone numbers of everyone associated with the center were stored in a computer located at Wieboldt Hall. Direct calls from outside bypassed the switchboard, eliminating heavy line traffic and avoiding long delays in reaching the desired extension. Any number within the center could be reached by dialing a four-digit extension.

Talking Computer Saves Time

A new computer was installed in radiation therapy that not only answered questions but asked them as well. This "talking computer" was connected to a teletypewriter, special TV screen and drawing board.

Using the teletype, a technician could "discuss" a case with the computer. On the TV screen, the computer might ask, "Where is the tumor?" and the operator would type the answer. Then, using the drawing board, the technician could "show" the computer the size of the tumor, proposed treatment and other information. When all of the computer's questions had been answered, it would indicate on the TV screen whether the treatment plan was appropriate.

The entire process of "computerized" dosimetry (measuring radioactivity) for one patient usually took only five to ten minutes. In the past, radiation technicians spent hours planning and calculating by hand the dosage and best position for treating various tumors. With the "talking" computer, the technician could give detailed study to 15 cases per day instead of three or four as in the past.

Emergency Capacity Extended

In the emergency department, an enlarged waiting room and additional examining rooms increased the area by half. Of great advantage to patients and Hospital alike were the new x-ray unit and attendant technicians in the emergency area itself, making it unnecessary to transport emergency patients to the third floor x-ray department.

Midwest Spinal Injury Care: Wesley and Rehabilitation Institute

In February, 1972, Wesley was designated by the Illinois Department of Public Health as a Special Regional Trauma Center for the care of patients with critical spinal cord injuries. An estimated 400 such cases occurred each year in Illinois. An emergency communication and transportation system was arranged to enable a person with a spinal cord injury to be brought from anywhere in Illinois to Wesley within four hours, the crucial time span to prevent irreversible cord damage, according to Dr. Paul R. Meyer, Jr., Wesley orthopedist and director of the center.

Although spinal injured patients could be treated elsewhere in Illinois, it was decided to place the activity within Northwestern's McGaw Medical Center for emergency and intensive care at Wesley, then long-term recovery at the nearly completed Rehabilitation Institute of Chicago, just half a block away.

Wesley's first acute spinal cord emergency case was David K. Bates, 18, who was injured in a digging accident in Simpson, Illinois, May 4, 1972. Doctors suspected spinal cord injury and notified the state's trauma network. Bates was flown by plane to Meigs field, then by helicopter to

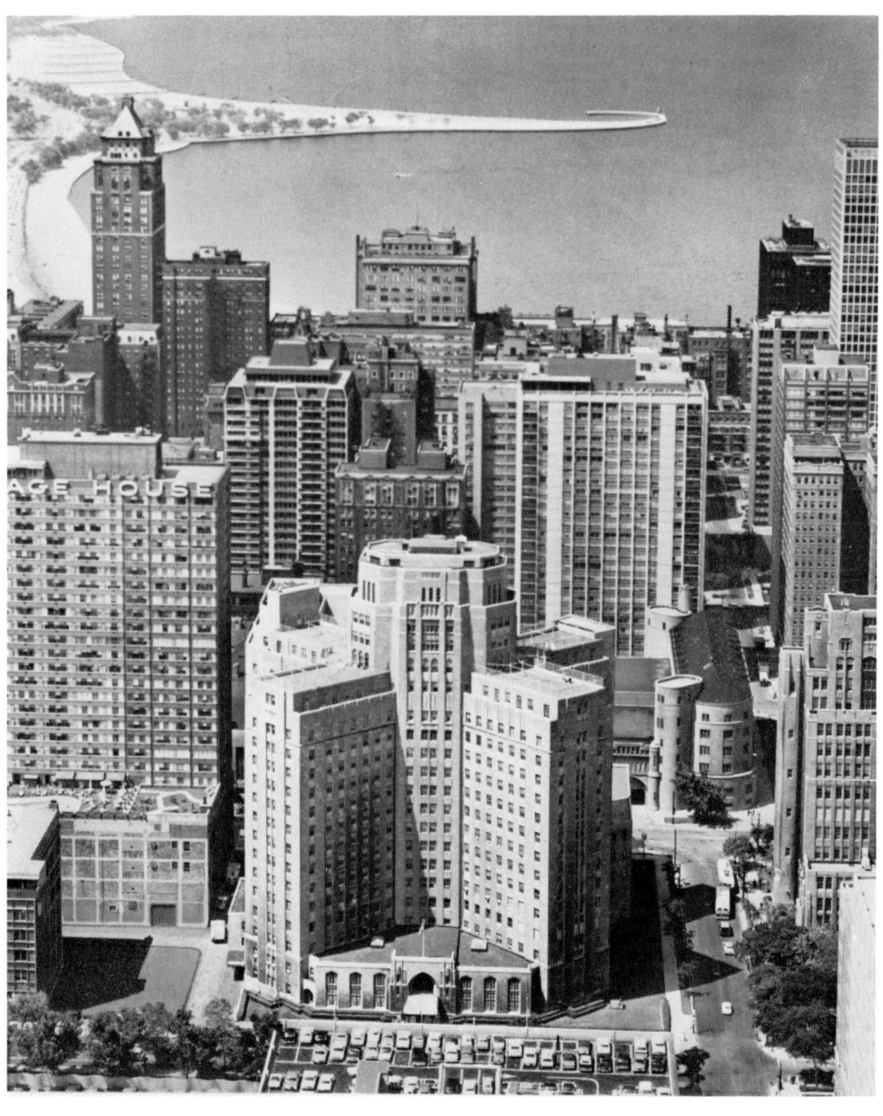

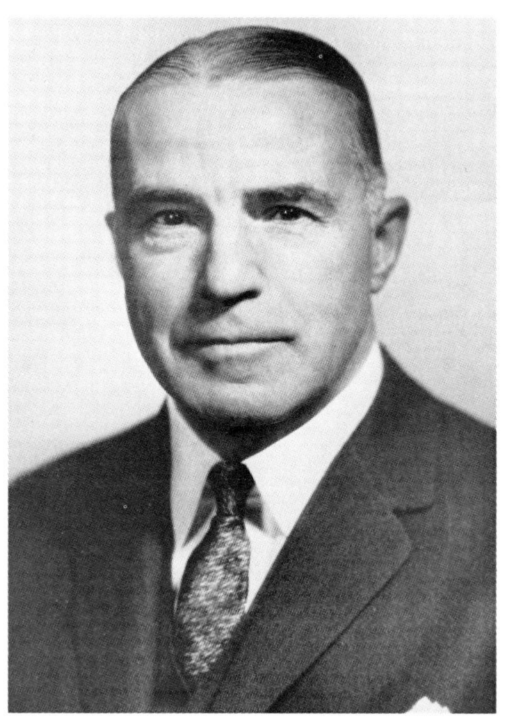

Thomas A. Harwood, elected trustee in 1940, served as president from 1961 until his death in 1964. His sound judgement helped the Wesley-Northwestern relationship.

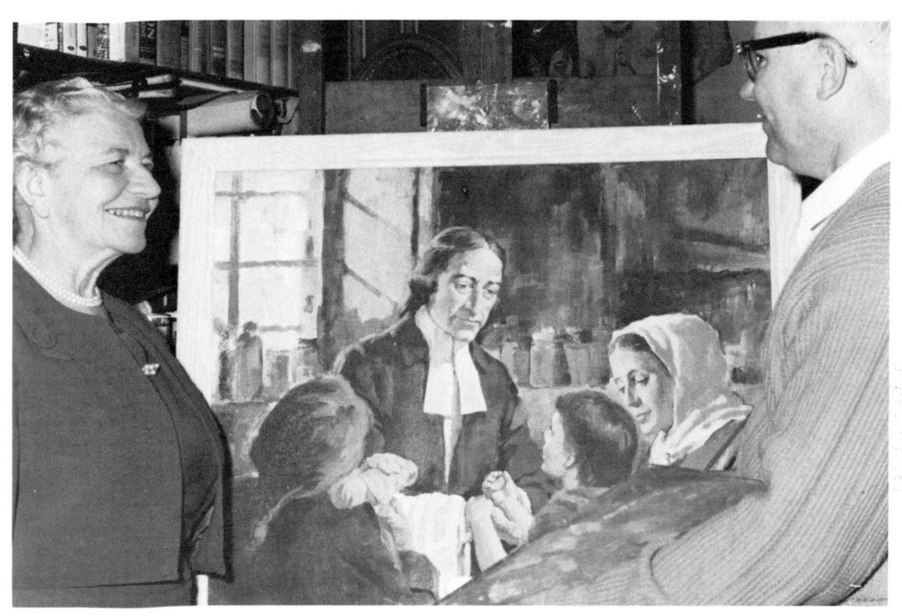

The painting, John Wesley, the Healer,
*the Auxiliary's memorial to Mr. Hardwood,
was viewed by Mrs. Charles Davis,
president, and John R. White, artist.*

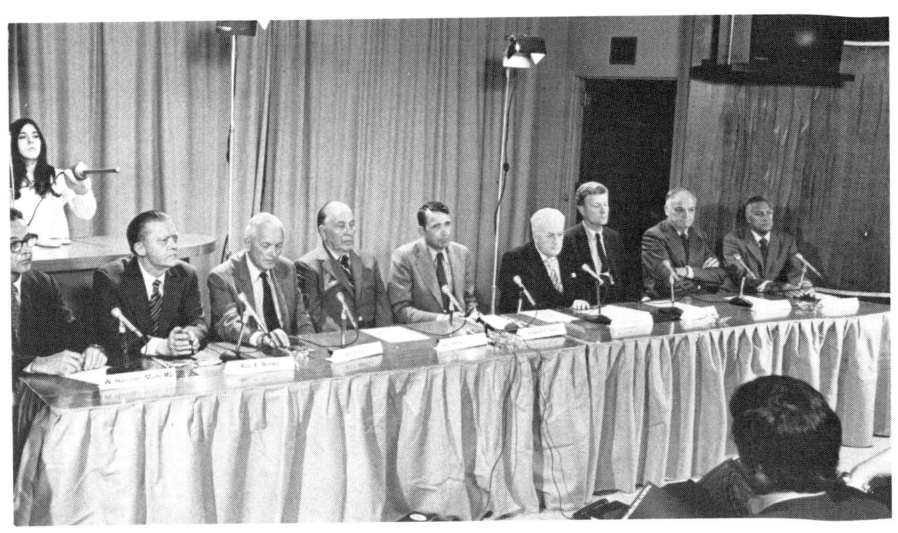

*Hospital, university and civic leaders
convened with press, August 15, 1972, to
announce the formation of Northwestern
Memorial Hospital.*

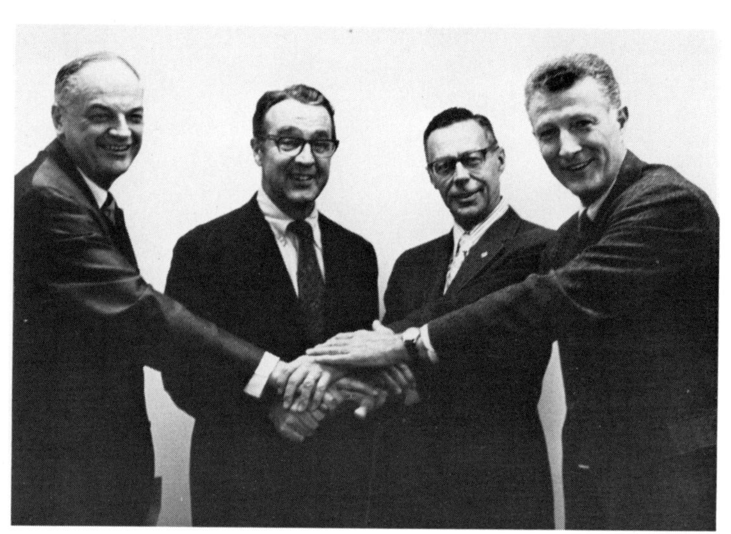

*Pledging teamwork: PMH president, John
Stagl; medical chief Harrison Mehn; CWMH
medical chief, Jacques Smith; president,
John Sturgis.*

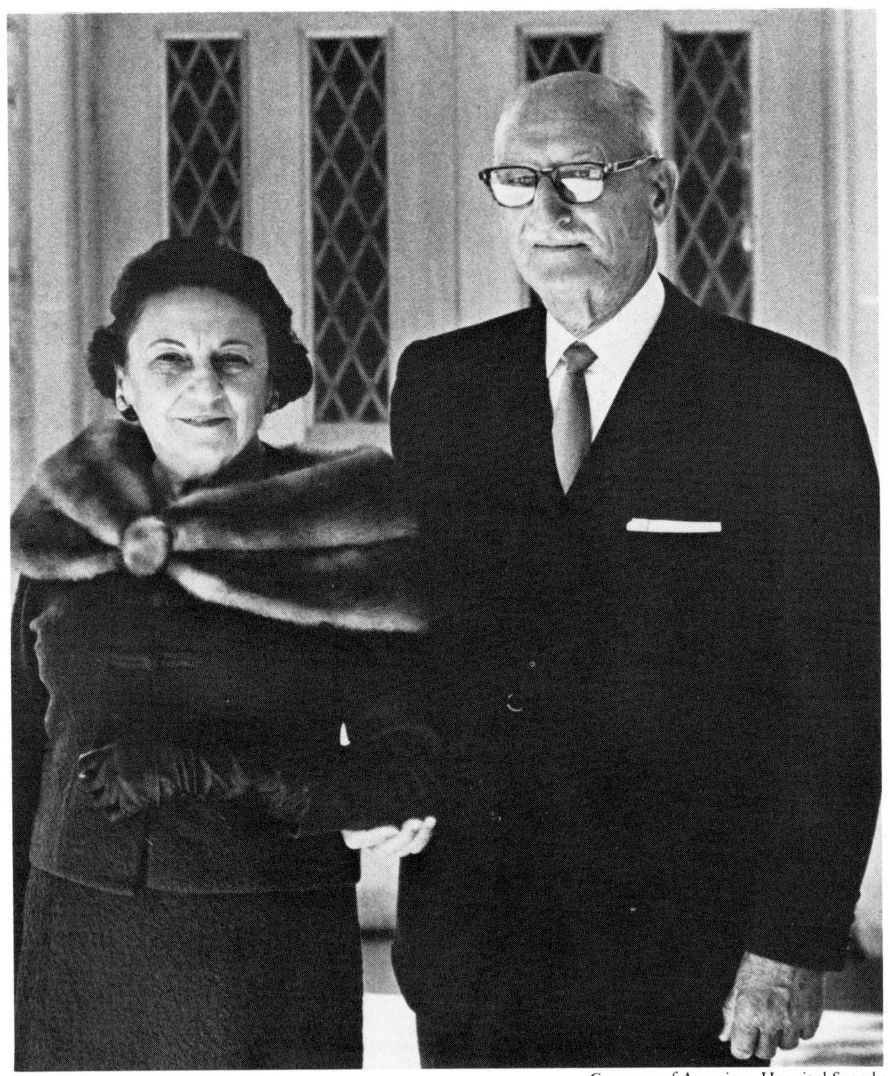

Courtesy of American Hospital Supply

Mary and Foster Glendale McGaw,
bounteous donors, who helped Wesley and
other NU affiliates through the McGaw
Medical Center of Northwestern University.

Lake Shore Park adjacent to Wesley. He was transported by stretcher to the emergency department where he received initial treatment, and then was admitted to the intensive care unit before transferral for rehabilitation.

In June the Department of Health, Education and Welfare approved a $1.5 million, five-year grant under the name of Midwest Regional Spinal Injury Care System (MRSICS) to be used in the acute spinal cord injury program specifically at Wesley and the Chicago Rehabilitation Institute.

ICCU Gives Continuity of Care

A six-bed intermediate coronary care unit (ICCU) was opened in July, 1972, for concentrated observation of patients with cardiovascular disease in the best possible environment for their recovery. The difference between the ICCU and the existing coronary care unit (CCU) was the type of cardiac monitoring. In CCU the monitors were attached to the patient by lead wires which confined the patient to bed. In ICCU the patient wore a small transistor device which transmitted the heart rhythm to the monitor by radio signals, a system called telemetry. It allowed the patient mobility so he could gradually begin to resume normal activity while still under observation. In ICCU, one monitor screen outside the patients' rooms displayed the heart rhythm patterns for six patients. In CCU a nurse had to remain in the patient's room to observe the monitor, so one nurse could care for only two patients. The major objective of the two units was to provide continuity of care for coronary patients requiring both types of surveillance during their recovery.

Rube Walker Leukemia Center

Wesley was a frequent recipient of gifts from sports fans who honored a player they admired by gifts to the hospital which had given him care. The Rube Walker Leukemia Center was dedicated in memory of Verlon (Rube) Walker, famous Chicago Cub coach and player, who had died of blood cancer at Wesley in March, 1971. A check for $35,000, representing the first gift to the Center, was presented by Cub first baseman, Ernie Banks, to purchase a Celltrifuge, white cell separator. In this device, a donor's blood was circulated continuously and, by centrifugal force, millions of normal white cells were harvested for the leukemia patient's use. The remainder of the blood, mainly red cells, was returned to the donor. The center consisted of two isolation rooms, equipped for intensive care, and a laboratory for personnel engaged in medical teaching and research. Dr. Wilson H. Hartz, Jr. was the director.

Hartman Retires Early

After nearly a quarter of a century of service to Wesley, Kenath Hartman, executive vice president, retired April 2, 1972. Although not yet of retirement age, he requested early retirement on advice of his doctors. He would remain on the Board of Trustees and continue to do volunteer work. Before joining Wesley in 1948, Hartman had spent a year as an administrative resident at Mt. Sinai Hospital in Chicago and six years in the United States Air Force. He considered that Wesley's most important events in which he played a major role were the merger of Wesley and Chicago Memorial hospitals in 1954, the expansion program which resulted in the Doctors Tower and Allison Pavilion in 1959, and the formation of the McGaw Medical Center of Northwestern University in 1969.

Wesley Doctor Named Teacher of 1972

Dr. Whitney Addington, director of Wesley's pulmonary function laboratory, was named "Outstanding Clinical Science Teacher of 1972" by the senior class of Northwestern Medical School at the May 20 NUMS alumni-faculty dinner. He was lauded by students as "the man who best demonstrated the fulfillment of the educational obligation of the practice of medicine." In addition to the pulmonary laboratory, Dr. Addington was director of Wesley's young adult cystic fibrosis clinic which recently had been accredited as a treatment center by the National Cystic Fibrosis Research Foundation. Dr. Addington was graduated from Princeton University and Northwestern University Medical School. He earned his master's degree from Oklahoma University.

Dr. Cannon Goes To Alaska

Dr. Abram Cannon, chairman of Wesley's diagnostic radiology department for more than 20 years, left July 1, 1972, to accept a position in a medical-surgical clinic in Fairbanks, Alaska. A graduate of Northwestern, Dr. Cannon was appointed radiology chairman at Wesley shortly after completing his residency in 1949. He directed diagnostic and therapeutic radiology until the latter became a separate department in 1956. His outstanding contributions were recognized at a dinner in his honor at the Lake Shore Club.

Four Corners Task Force Aim: Better Care for More People

A task force was formed in late 1971, spearheaded by Ray E. Brown, executive vice president of the McGaw Medical Center of Northwestern University. Its purpose was to study ways to smooth the flow of medical care between the center members—Wesley, Passavant, and the medical school—located at the geographic four corners of the Superior Street-Fairbanks Court intersection. It was recognized that pooling certain services and facilities in both clinical and operational areas between the two hospitals would provide superior services more efficiently to more people.

The Four Corners Task Force consisted of representatives from the major medical services and administrators from Wesley and Passavant hospitals, Northwestern University Medical School, and the McGaw Medical Center. The Task Force was charged to take a thorough look at the physical plants, land ownership of each, professional services then offered, the patient load and projected future needs.

It went without saying that all long-range development programs of Wesley and Passavant were set aside until the Task Force report, due January, 1972, became available. Cooperative measures begun or scheduled almost immediately were increased group purchasing, centralized laboratories and computers, shared respiratory therapy, and emergency service. The Four Corners Task Force made about 30 recommendations to synchronize service at Wesley and Passavant hospitals, paving the way for total consolidation.

The President Expresses His Hopes

The May, 1972, issue of *Wesley MEMO*, the monthly publication for employees and friends, featured an interview between the editor, Jeff Gerew, and Wesley President John C. Sturgis. Excerpts follow:

Memo: You've been here a year and a half; what do you feel have been some of your accomplishments in that time?

Sturgis: . . . I suppose the first thing is taking advantage of some fine old ideas around here which have never been brought off. The first of these was the open staff agreement between us and Passavant. Oddly enough, most people don't know, or have forgotten, that this idea was the original intention when the present building was opened 31 years ago.

Secondly, I recognize that, more than anyone else, I am responsible for stopping the building of the western addition to Wesley. I continue to believe that this is a "B" plan . . . The "A" plan is a building which brings together Wesley, Passavant and Northwestern Medical School, and that's the plan we are working toward. Hopefully, we will have a new building[1] on the parking lot at Fairbanks and Superior corners within the next four years.

Memo: Presumably, this is all tied in with the recent merger study approved by Wesley's and Passavant's trustees.

Sturgis: Yes. Our real dream is a great medical center. We have the medical staffs, history, location, trustees, access to money, and great university connection. We're not missing anything except putting it all together.

Memo: In the past, Wesley's relationship with the Medical School hasn't been the best. Would you comment on this?

Sturgis: . . . I know there has been aggravation in the past, some of it real and some of it imagined . . . I think, though, in the last several years, there has been a noticeable diminution of this type of aggravation.

Memo: Why do you believe this is now true?

Sturgis: Primarily because the people in leadership positions have changed, and with those changes have come people who recognize the growing magnitude of the problem of delivering health care. It's so enormous that we really haven't time anymore to take on each other in meaningless vendettas, but must get on with the problem of attacking the real enemy which is the great gap between health care needed and health care available.

Memo: Is Wesley loosening its ties with the Methodist Church?

Sturgis: . . . I think you have to find out first what those ties really were. Certainly, the Methodist Church must be given full credit for the establishment of the hospital. On the other hand, I gather the rather low financial support of Wesley by the Methodist Church is based on the belief that the hospital has the power and ability to obtain funds on its own. They are directing funds to efforts which are probably not as able to get their own funds as Wesley is . . .

---

[1]*Mr. Sturgis' hopeful prophecy became a reality when the Health Sciences Building was dedicated October 8, 1979.*

And finally...Consolidation　　Chapter 27

S lowly, deliberately, Wesley and Passavant advanced through the latter part of the sixtieth decade as neighbors whose single purpose, excellence of health care, guided them in one direction only— consolidation into a modern major medical center hospital.

MARVELOUS MESHINGS

It started with the doctors, as did Wesley itself, seeking the best way to treat their patients with the available facilities. Even before the formation of the Northwestern University Medical Center in 1966, certain measures pointed to cooperation. For instance, the Wesley medical staff revised its bylaws to permit a member to join the staff of another affiliated hospital. Increased group buying reaped greater savings. Such actions, both operational and clinical, were accelerated by early recommendations of the Four Corners Task Force. Only Wesley offered radiation therapy; Passavant alone had hemodialysis. All neurosurgery was performed in Wesley's ultramodern suite; all eye surgery was conducted at Passavant, where precision instruments included an argon laser photocoagulator. Wesley psychiatrists found they had a waiting list in March, 1971; Passavant's mental health floor had empty beds. They decided to exchange privileges to equalize occupancy, avoid delays and expedite care. Five months later the entire medical staffs of both Wesley and Passavant hospitals voted for reciprocal privileges. Each could admit patients, write orders and use all facilities at the other hospital. Describing the intense period of partial consolidations, shared services and coordinated efforts, Dr. Melvyn A. Bayly, Wesley's immediate past chief of staff, called it "one of the most marvelous meshings of medical mechanisms."

Wesley-Passavant Nursing Schools Unite

The first segment of Wesley and Passavant to combine completely was nursing education. The joining together of Wesley's School of Nursing, founded in 1889, and of Passavant's James Ward Thorne School of Nursing, founded in 1898[1], was announced April 11, 1972, by the two Northwestern-affiliated hospitals. The merged school would become the largest hospital-affiliated nursing education program in the Midwest. Wesley's current enrollment was 247 and Passavant's was 92, a total of 339 which was expected to reach 360 by September, 1973.

Wesley President John C. Sturgis explained "the September, 1972, freshman class and subsequent classes should eventually result in an annual saving of approximately $200,000." The facilities at both hospitals would continue to be used for the students' clinical experience. The freshman class would live at Passavant's Worcester House and the juniors and seniors at Wesley's Carriage House.

Wesley Women Form New Board

In preparation for coming events, a Woman's Board was formed in April of five Wesley volunteer groups represented by a volunteer council. The board's first president was Hester S. Doughty, a volunteer with more than 1,500 service hours. As president of the Woman's Board, Mrs. Doughty would serve on Wesley's Board of Trustees.

Also elected were Francis L. Morris, 1st vice president, volunteer director of the patient library; Alice Walker Bowles, 2nd vice president, 1st vice president of the service league; Demetra Svolos, corresponding secretary, an inservice volunteer; Elaine H. Markus, recording secretary, volunteer and staff nurse in the obstetrical department, and Mildred B. Gerk, treasurer, newsletter editor for the woman's auxiliary.

Although each of the five groups, the woman's auxiliary, service league,

[1]*The original Passavant nursing school was suspended in 1935 and re-established in 1949 through Mrs. James Ward Thorne.*

volunteers, patients' library and nurse alumnae, voted for ultimate unity, each would retain its individual projects. The 1971 outgoing president of the service league, Mrs. Edward L. Compere, presented checks for $145,000, contributed during her tenure, for improvements at Wesley.

SHALL WE MERGE?

Back in the early thirties, ten years before Wesley moved to its near north location, the two hospitals had considered joining together. Minutes of the Wesley trustee executive committee meeting June 30, 1931, reported that, regarding meetings with Passavant directors relative to merger with Passavant Hospital, not much progress was made. "There were many things of grave import to be decided before the wisdom of such a step could be determined."

The second time around, more than forty years later, a special consolidation study committee was formed May 3, 1972, to investigate the "many things of grave import." The committee was charged by the Wesley and Passavant governing boards to make a formal feasibility study starting June 5, 1972, of the proposed merger. It was comprised of ten members from each hospital's board, medical staff and administration. Representing Wesley were Drs. Leon A. Carrow and Jacques M. Smith; Messrs. T. Stanton Armour, William B. Browder, Henry Gardner, Hubert E. Howard, Jr., Peter H. Merlin, John C. Sturgis, Edward F. Swift, and Gordon Worley. Representing Passavant were Drs. William A. Larmon and W. Harrison Mehn; Messrs. H. Templeton Brown, Robert M. Buddington, Silas S. Cathcart, Edison Dick, John S. Hutchins, Gilbert H. Scribner, Jr., John M. Stagl, and Edwin A. Steubner.

Five sub-committees were appointed to study the benefits of consolidation: financial affairs, legal, personnel, organization management and medical affairs. The consolidation committee was expected to present its recommendations at the August board meetings of both hospitals. Discussing the study, Wesley Chairman Edward F. Swift commented: "The advantages of joint effort have become increasingly obvious. The question to be resolved by the study is whether or not it best serves the interest of our patients and community that we extend this effort to a total merger.

"Certainly, the potential is great. A merger would result in a university-affiliated, teaching and research hospital, equivalent in size and expertise to any other hospital or medical center in the Midwest. It would ideally combine the best of both present institutions."

CONSOLIDATION IS APPROVED

A majority of Wesley's Board of Trustees met in the Presidents' Room of the University Club of Chicago at the regular August meeting and approved a nine-page Plan and Agreement of Consolidation from which the following is excerpted:

WITNESSETH:

WHEREAS, each of the parties deems it advisable for its general welfare and advantage that both parties be consolidated into a single new corporation, and respectively desire to effect such consolidation pursuant to this Agreement and the applicable provisions of the General Not For Profit Corporation Act of the State of Illinois;

NOW, THEREFORE, in consideration of the premises and of the mutual agreements and undertakings herein contained, the parties hereto hereby agree to consolidate, and to do all acts or things necessary or desirable to effectuate the same...

PLAN OF CONSOLIDATION

Chicago Wesley Memorial Hospital and Passavant Memorial Hospital (said corporations being hereinafter collectively referred to as the "Constituent Corporations") shall be consolidated into a single new corporation, to wit: NORTHWESTERN MEMORIAL HOSPITAL (hereinafter called the "Resulting Corporation") which shall exist under and be governed by the provisions of the General Not For Profit Corporation Act of the State of Illinois...

EFFECT OF CONSOLIDATION

When the consolidation has been effected the separate existence of the Constituent Corporations shall cease. The Resulting Corporation shall thereupon and thereafter possess all the rights, privileges, immunities and franchises of each of the Constituent Corporations...

The purposes for which the corporation is organized are:
(i) to establish and maintain institutions which provide comprehensive health services to the sick and injured;
(ii) to provide medical educational programs;
(iii) to encourage research and ways to save human life, minimize human suffering, and improve health services; and
(iv) to mobilize all community support and resources to serve the comprehensive health needs of the corporation's community...

The corporation is organized exclusively for charitable, scientific and educational purposes as a not for profit corporation, and its activities shall be conducted for the aforesaid purposes in such a manner that no part of its net earnings shall inure to the benefit of any member, director, officer or individual. Upon dissolution of the corporation, and after payment of just debts and liabilities, all remaining assets shall be distributed to organizations enjoying an exempt status under section 501 (c) (3) of the Internal Revenue Code of 1954, as amended, or successor provisions. The corporation shall not substantially engage in carrying on propaganda or otherwise attempting to influence legislation...

WESLEY + PASSAVANT = NORTHWESTERN MEMORIAL HOSPITAL

Announcement of the consolidation was made at a press conference the following day at Passavant's Offield Auditorium, attended by Mayor Richard J. Daley and representatives of both hospitals, Northwestern University and the McGaw Medical Center of Northwestern University. The new Northwestern Memorial Hospital had nearly 1,000 beds (Wesley had 615 beds; Passavant, 378) and was the largest private hospital in the State of Illinois.

Wesley's board chairman, Edward F. Swift III, became chairman of the Board of Directors of Northwestern Memorial Hospital and Passavant's board chairman, John S. Hutchins, was named vice chairman. John C. Sturgis, president of Wesley, was chairman of the new board's executive committee, and John M. Stagl, president of Passavant, was president and chief operating officer of the new hospital.

Northwestern Memorial had 79 members on its Board of Directors composed of Wesley's 44 trustees and Passavant's 35 directors. Wesley's 1,685 employees and Passavant's 858 employees totaled 2,543 for Northwestern Memorial. The combined medical staff numbered 450 doctors. The names of the original hospitals were retained as pavilions: the Wesley Pavilion and Passavant Pavilion.

ACCORDING TO THE PAPERS...

Chicago newspapers were generous in praise of the two hospitals they knew so well, both as news sources and, because of proximity, as personal health facilities in times of illness. The following excerpts are printed with permission from the newspapers.

Education was stressed

The merger of Wesley Memorial and Passavant Memorial Hospitals into Northwestern Memorial Hospital can only add to Chicago's recognized greatness as a medical teaching center. Both are affiliated with Northwestern University Medical School and the combined institution will have a new strength and flexibility...

Yet Chicago because of its medical richness, can afford to throw off binding tradition and move with awareness and purpose to bring community health needs and medical education together. Much is being done, but there is an infinite amount more to do, and the burden rests upon all the city's medical institutions, from the oldest to the newest.

Editorial page of the Chicago Sun-Times, August 17, 1972.

They focused on finances

As patients know all too well, hospital costs are soaring out of sight. Anything that can be done to hold the line while continuing to keep up with the advance of medical science serves the interests of both the patients and the donors whose gifts must help sustain the private hospitals...

The financial benefits can be considerable. In nearly every medical specialty, the array of technical equipment available is increasing in variety and in cost. A single cardiac surgery unit or neurological center, for example, can serve both hospitals without costly duplication in each. Physicians and surgeons can combine their skills in specialized centers that complement each other instead of competing...

Editorial page of the Chicago Daily News, August 16, 1972.

Predicted better patient care

...Ray E. Brown, executive vice president of the Northwestern University-McGaw Medical Center, stated last spring, "The notion of merger is based on the potential of reduced overhead, elimination of duplicated services and facilities, opportunities for new and expanded programs, and the improved economy and quality that accompany increased scale."

...Both hospitals have seen and grasped an opportunity "to provide better patient care at a reduced cost," to quote the president of the Passavant board, John S. Hutchins...

More a marriage than a merger

...The full merger involves little visible sacrifice except of sentimental attachments to the honorable separate records, past and present, of Wesley and Passavant. Recognition that this merger is more like a marriage than like a merger of business competitors should assuage such pangs.

Chicago Tribune, August 16, 1972

Doctors were commended

By unanimously supporting the merger of Chicago Wesley Memorial and Passavant Memorial Hospitals, doctors at the two institutions have moved a new landmark into the field of medical education. Consolidating two hospitals, each with separate departments, department heads, power bases and interests, is not an easy task. It's to the credit of the medical staffs that they put self-interest aside to accept the larger goals of improved medical education and patient care.

Northwestern Memorial Hospital, as the new combined institution will be called, will double the number of cases available to interns and residents and considerably increase their learning experience; and aside from the obvious financial savings which will accrue to the hospitals from consolidating their administration, the real advantage of the merger lies in improved health care for Chicagoans.

The creation of a new, high-prestige teaching institution, in the center of the vital Northwestern University-McGaw Medical Center, can only bode well for the health of both the city and its residents.

Editorial, Chicago Tribune, August 18, 1972

Epilogue

In retrospect, the consolidation of Chicago Wesley Memorial and Passavant Memorial hospitals was inevitable. The subject had been discussed ten years before Wesley joined Passavant on Northwestern University's Chicago campus, had been recorded in the Wesley Board of Trustees minutes in 1931, then tabled for forty years.

Meanwhile Wesley grew through gifts of property and endowment plus two major mergers which provided instant medical staff, personnel and additional financial assets. Wesley was founded by a physician in 1888 under the aegis of the Methodist Church which gave limited sustained maintenance and a broad base of volunteers. The bylaws stipulated that three-fourths of the board be members of the Methodist Church and most donors were of that faith. While they were forward-looking men and women, they also were conservative. They viewed teaching innovations of the Northwestern University Medical School, with which Wesley was affiliated, with more pragmatism than optimism for nearly thirty years. Finally a compromise was reached that could, and eventually did, result in amicable cooperation.

Passavant, on the other hand, had grown from the inside out, with no acquisitions other than gifts from affluent friends and members of the Board of Directors. It was founded in 1865 by a Lutheran clergyman and, like Wesley, its first nurses were trained Deaconesses following the precepts of the early Christian church. Passavant had burned to the ground in the Chicago Fire of 1871, and had risen again after 14 years, a stronger, better hospital, continuing to care for the sick until 1925 when it closed because of obsolete facilities.

In 1921, Northwestern University, then involved in a "Greater Northwestern" program to build schools of Medicine, Dentistry, Law and Commerce at recently acquired property on Chicago's near north side, invited Passavant to affiliate and move to the new campus. However, the old question, "Who selects physicians on the hospital staff?" delayed action (as it did at Wesley) until 1925 when a compromise satisfactory to both the university and Passavant was reached.

On May 21, 1929, Passavant dedicated its new building diagonally across the street from property that Northwestern University still reserved for Wesley. Twelve years later Wesley joined its co-affiliate on the Northwestern campus. Hence the neighboring hospitals, with similar lineage and heritage, proceeded with their identical purposes: healing the sick and training doctors for the future.

Thus Wesley, in its ninety-third year, united with its natural partner, Passavant, to become Northwestern Memorial Hospital, and perform health services for humanity that neither could achieve alone.

The three essential components of a hospital—compassion, medical science and facilities—abound at the new institution. Patients are accorded personalized compassionate care by nurses and other trained personnel whose respect for human dignity is inherent to their calling. Physicians augment medical science, gleaned from the past, with today's exciting research findings enabling them to improve and lengthen life. The constantly updated precision equipment and appropriate patient accommodations aid the doctor in performing modern medical miracles.

Wesley and Passavant hospitals accumulated separately the equivalent of two centuries of medical experience within their walls. Their combined strength along with that of the Institute of Psychiatry, Prentice Women's Hospital and Maternity Center, and the Olson Critical Care Pavilion, now is embodied in Northwestern Memorial Hospital which contributes mightily to the total health environment of the McGaw Medical Center of Northwestern University. Here, in the last quarter of the 20th century, may be found the realization of Hippocrates' precept voiced during the fourth century B.C.: "Where there is love for mankind, there is love for the art of healing."[1]

[1]*Address by Donald J. Caseley, M.D., vice chancellor emeritus, University of Illinois, June 1980, unveiling a sculpture of Hippocrates.*

Appendix

PRESIDENTS OF THE BOARD OF TRUSTEES
Wesley Hospital, Wesley Memorial Hospital, Chicago Wesley Memorial Hospital

PRESIDENTS OF THE WOMEN'S AUXILIARY

Mrs. Bishop O. Lovejoy, 1937-1946
Mrs. Oliver R. Aspegren, 1946-1949
Mrs. Edward J. Smerz, 1949-1951
Mrs. Arthur L. Myers, 1951-1954
Mrs. Richard G. Breeden, 1954-1956
Mrs. Charles Randolph, 1956-1960

Mrs. Andrew S. Hurter, 1960-1963
Mrs. Jesse L. Blaine, 1963-1965
Mrs. Winfield W. Scott, 1965-1966
Mrs. Jesse L. Blaine, 1966-1967
Mrs. Charles F. Davis, 1967-1971
Mrs. William V. Willcox, 1971-1972

PRESIDENTS OF THE SERVICE LEAGUE

Mrs. Felix Jansey, 1935-1942
Mrs. Gilbert H. Marquardt, 1943
Mrs. Gerard N. Krost, 1943-1944
Mrs. Harry M. Richter, 1945-1946
Mrs. Blanche D. Carr, 1947-1949
Mrs. Munro Maddock, 1949-1951
Mrs. John Spry Holmes, 1951-1953
Mrs. Robert J. Giltnane, 1953-1954
Mrs. Francis D. Wolfe, 1954-1956

Mrs. Edward M. Dorr, 1957-1958
Mrs. George H. Gardner, 1958-1960
Mrs. Ronald R. Greene, 1960-1962
Mrs. Edward L. Compere, 1962-1964
Mrs. Jack A. Handley, 1964-1966
Mrs. William A. Mann, 1966-1968
Mrs. Edward L. Compere, 1969-1970
Mrs. Maxwell Mulmat, 1971-1972

ADMINISTRATIVE STAFF
August, 1971

John C. Sturgis
President

Kenath Hartman
Executive Vice President

Marlin J. Barklage
Vice President, Personnel

Donald A. Bloom
Vice President, Administration

Ronald D. Olmsted
*Vice President, Development and
Public Relations*

Harold J. Staidl
Vice President, Finance

Vera E. Thompson
*Vice President, Nursing Care and
Nursing Education*

Anne B. Blanton
Assistant Vice President

William R. Mumma
*Assistant Vice President, Administration;
Director, Food Services*

Kenneth Overly
*Assistant Vice President, Administration;
Director, Occupational Therapy*

Michael F. Alexa
Director, Patient Service Coordination

James A. Angstrom
Manager, Laundry

Virginia Barlow
Manager, Telephone Communications

Arnie F. Betts
Director, Public Relations

Dorothy Blott
Director, Volunteers

The Rev. Robert A. Dahl
Chaplain

Frances Dreyer
Manager, Internal Auditing

Andrew G. Fallat
Administrative Resident

Frank Gagarin
Staff Architect

Rhodora Hopkins
Administrative Assistant, Evenings

Robert Hurley
Director, Security

Ronald T. Maiter
Director, Materials Management

John H. Martin
Director, Housekeeping

Joseph M. Mathews
Director, Patient Financial Services

Donald M. Michels
Director, Management Information Service

Kenneth R. Miller
Director, Development

Joseph Palukas
Manager, Cost and Insurance

Lucille Plotke
Manager, Admitting

Robert E. Sweeney
Manager, Carriage House

June M. Wallace
Director, Medical Records

William V. Willcox
Comptroller

CHIEF EXECUTIVE OFFICERS

The Reverend Josiah Shelley Meyer,
   1888-1892
The Reverend George Jeffrey,
   1892-1893
The Reverend Joseph Odgers,
   1893-1895
Joseph S. Harvey, 1895-1898
The Reverend Josiah Shelley Meyer,
   1898-1901

A. Dudley Jackson, M.D., 1901-1908
Eugene S. Gilmore, 1908-1931
Paul H. Fesler, 1931-1936
Ernest R. Snyder, 1936-1939
Raymond W. McNealy, M.D.,
   1940-1942
Edgar Blake, Jr., 1942-1947
Ralph M. Hueston, 1947-1959
Kenath Hartman, 1960-1972

PROFESSIONAL SERVICES STAFF
August, 1971

Maxine Brewer
Administrative Assistant, Pathology

Lois Ebinger
Director, Nursing Education

Mary Emanuelson
Director, Social Work

Dorothea L. Fee
Director, Nursing Service

Lee Gladstone, M.D.
*Medical Director, Psychiatric Day
Hospital*

Ann Grant
Administrative Assistant, Anesthesiology

Emma L. Grimm
Associate Director, Nursing Service

Ben T. Howiler
Director, Pharmacy

John R. Hughes, Ph.D.
Medical Director, Electroencephalography

Raja K. Khuri, **M**.D.
Medical Director, Health Services

Robert T. Marshall, M.D.
Medical Director, Research Services

Sheridan Meyers, M.D.
Medical Director, Heart Station

Earliene Mitchler
Administrative Assistant, Diagnostic Radiology

Mary Morton
Director, Physical Therapy

James L. Quinn, III, M.D.
Medical Director, Nuclear Medicine

Bernice M. Sexauer
Executive Dietitian

Barry A. Shapiro, M.D.
Medical Director, Respiratory Therapy

Carol Trout, RN, A.R.I.T.
Director, Respiratory Therapy

MEDICAL STAFF
August 31, 1971

*Anesthesia and
Inhalation Therapy*

Edward A. Brunner, M.D.,
Chairman

Attending:
John W. Ditzler, M.D.
James E. Eckenhoff, M.D.

Associate Attending:
Lawrence M. Berman, M.D.
Edward A. Brunner, M.D.
Lawrence S. Chun, M.D.
Paul E. Hodel, M.D.
Jack Kamen, M.D.
Verner E. Lamb, M.D.
John D. Leahy, M.D.
Carolyn Wilkinson, M.D.
Lawrence Wilson, M.D.

Adjunct
James Gildea, M.D.
William Gottschalk, M.D.

John Homi, M.D.
Ronald Kilzer, M.D.
Frank Raymon, M.D.
Ann Ronai, M.D.
Barry Shapiro, M.D.
James C. Rich, M.D.
Sang Ho Yuo, M.D.

Affiliated Professional Staff

Consultant:
David Bruce, M.D.

Associate Staff:
Harry W. Linde, Ph.D.

Dermatology
Samuel M. Bluefarb, M.D.,
Chairman

Attending:
Samuel M. Bluefarb, M.D.

Associate Attending:
William A. Caro, M.D.
Ruth Freinkel, M.D.
Fred Levit, M.D.

Rocco A. Masessa, M.D.
Beatrice E. Tucker, M.D.

Associate Attending:
Robert Bouer, M.D.
Samuel Edwards, M.D.
Richard Elesh, M.D.
Jerome D. Kaufman, M.D.
Richard K. Luke, M.D.
Barton I. Mann, M.D.
Raymond A. McDermott, Jr., M.D.

Adjunct:
John J. Barton, M.D.
Donald R. Dye, M.D.
Leonard Rapoport, M.D.

Affiliated Professional Staff

Consultant:
Ronald Greene, M.D.

Ophthalmology
Earl H. Merz, M.D.,
Chairman
William A. Mann, M.D.,
Chairman Emeritus

Attending:
James G. Dobbie, M.D.
Orville E. Gordon, M.D.
Helen Holt, M.D.
William A. Mann, M.D.
Earl H. Merz, M.D.
Robert G. Miller, M.D.
Richard A. Perritt, M.D.
Kenneth L. Roper, M.D.

Associate Attending:
Curtis F. Deters, M.D.
Seymour B. Goren, M.D.
Joel Sacks, M.D.

Orthopedic Surgery
William J. Kane, M.D.,
Chairman

Edward L. Compere, M.D.,
Chairman Emeritus

Attending:
Robert G. Addison, M.D.
Sam W. Banks, M.D.
Clinton L. Compere, M.D.
Edward L. Compere, M.D.
William B. Fischer, M.D.
William Kane, M.D.
Hampar Kelikian, M.D.
William J. Schnute, M.D.
Robert G. Thompson, M.D.

Associate Attending:
Jerome R. Head, Jr., M.D.
Robert D. Keagy, M.D.
William T. Kernahan, Jr., M.D.
Paul R. Meyer, Jr., M.D.
Shahan K. Sarrafian, M.D.
Mihran O. Tachdjian, M.D.

*Otolaryngology and
Maxillofacial Surgery*
George A. Sisson, M.D.,
Chairman

Attending:
George W. Allen, M.D.
Richard P. Ariagno, M.D.
Eugene L. Derlacki, M.D.
Wiley H. Harrison, M.D.
Gordon H. Scott, M.D.
Goerge E. Shambaugh, Jr., M.D.
George A. Sisson, M.D.
Ira J. Tresley, M.D.

Associate Attending:
Jerome Goldstein, M.D.
Jack D. Kerth, M.D.

Dental Staff:
Dale Clark, DDS

Adjunct Dental Staff:
Thomas E. Cummings, DDS
Leon Rosenfeld, DDS

Affiliated Professional Staff
Consultant:
Cecil Hart, M.D.

Associate Staff:
Malcolm Hast, Ph.D.

Pathology
Geoffrey Kent, M.D.,
Chairman

Attending:
Frank R. Carone, M.D.
Geoffrey Kent, M.D.
Kenneth A. Schneider, M.D.

Associate Attending:
Phillip Barney, M.D.
Hector Battifora, M.D.
Jan Leestma, M.D.
Roy T. Smith, M.D.
Boyd O. Wilson, M.D.

Associate Visiting Staff:
Herbert M. Sommers, M.D.

Adjunct Visiting Staff:
Hsiang Mei Liu, M.D.

Affiliated Professional Staff
Consultant:
Robert B. Jennings, M.D.

Associate Staff:
Alan Chakrin, Ph.D.
Edward J. Fitzsimons, Ph.D.
Benny C. Jee, Ph.D.

Pediatrics
John J. Boehm, M.D.,
Chairman

Attending:
John P. Andrews, M.D.
Edward Beasley, M.D.
L. Martin Hardy, M.D.
Edmond R. Hess, M.D.
Gerard N. Krost, M.D.
Robert B. Lawson, M.D.
Eugene L. Slotkowski, M.D.
William W. Swanson, M.D.
Vida B. Wentz, M.D.
Elsie I. Wieczorowski, M.D.

Associate Attending:
John J. Boehm, M.D.
Harold Goodman, M.D.
Eloise E. Johnson, M.D.
Laurel E. Keith, M.D.
James Nicklas, M.D.
Oscar A. Novick, M.D.
Howard S. Traisman, M.D.

Adjunct:
Howard Rice, M.D.

Psychiatry
Harold M. Visotsky, M.D.,
Chairman

Attending:
Benjamin Blackman, M.D.
Benjamin Boshes, M.D.
John W. Lauer, M.D.
William B. Spriegel, M.D.
Harold M. Visotsky, M.D.

Associate Attending:
Nelson Borelli, M.D.
Rolando E. de la Torre, M.D.
R. Patricia Field, M.D.
Ronald Shlensky, M.D.
Lowell C. Wigdahl, M.D.

Adjunct:
Richard Abrams, M.D.

Harry M. Charkatz, M.D.
Lee Gladstone, M.D.
Richard Rappaport, M.D.

Affiliated Professional Staff

Associate Staff:
Jack Arbit, Ph.D.
Nathaniel Raskin, Ph.D.
Micha Zaks, Ph.D.

Surgery

James R. Hines, M.D.,
Chairman

Attending:
John M. Beal, M.D.
John J. Bergan, M.D.
Arthur DeBoer, M.D.
Samuel J. Fogelson, M.D.
Robert E. Geurkink, M.D.
Michael C. Govostis, M.D.
B. Herold Griffith, M.D.
Jerome R. Head, Sr., M.D.
Richard E. Heller, M.D.
William A. Hendricks, M.D.
James R. Hines, M.D.
Raymond Householder, M.D.
Theodore R. Hudson, M.D.
Felix Jansey, M.D.
Earl O. Latimer, M.D.
William M. McMillan, M.D.
Norman G. Parry, M.D.
Peter A. Rosi, M.D.
Durand Smith, M.D.

Associate Attending:
William L. Donnellan, M.D.
Lester E. Garrison, M.D.
Louis R. Head, M.D.
Gabriel Lorenzo, M.D.
Peter W. McKinney, M.D.
Frederick W. Preston, M.D.
William M. Walker, M.D.

Adjunct:
Frederick K. Merkel, M.D.
Fred M. Miller, M.D.
Thomas Murphy, M.D.
Leo R. Radigan, M.D.
Charles J. Staley, M.D.
Otto H. Trippel, M.D.
Gerald Ujicki, M.D.
Robert M. Vanecko, M.D.
Walter N. Wiborg, M.D.

Affiliated Professional Staff

Visiting:
Thomas Shields, M.D.

Consultant:
T. Howard Clarke, M.D.

Therapeutic Radiology

William T. Moss, M.D.,
Chairman

Attending:
William T. Moss, M.D.
James L. Quinn, III, M.D.

Associate Attending:
William Brand, M.D.

Adjunct:
Gerald G. Beck, M.D.

Affiliated Professional Staff

Associate Staff:
Warren McGonnagle, Ph.D.
Bryan R. Westerman, Ph.D.

Urology

Vincent J. O'Conor, Jr., M.D.,
Chairman

Attending:
George J. Bulkley, M.D.
Andrew McNally, Jr., M.D.
Vincent J. O'Conor, Jr., M.D.
J. Kenneth Sokol, M.D.

Adjunct:
John B. Nanninga, M.D.

Affiliated Professional Staff

Consultant:
John T. Grayhack, M.D.

CHIEFS OF STAFF

Weller Van Hook, M.D., 1900-1905
Thomas J. Watkins, M.D., 1906-1912
William E. Schroeder, M.D., 1912-1926
Charles A. Elliott, M.D., 1926-1927
Allan B. Kanavel, M.D., 1928
J. Gordon Wilson, M.D., 1929
William H. Holmes, M.D., 1930-1931
Charles B. Reed, M.D., 1932-34
Mark T. Goldstine, M.D., 1935-1936
Robert Blue, M.D., 1937-1938
Raymond W. McNealy, M.D., 1939-1940
William Miller, M.D., 1941
Gilbert H. Marquardt, M.D., 1941-42 1946-47

Gerard N. Krost, M.D., 1942-44
Paul G. Rhoads, M.D., 1945
Vincent J. O'Conor, M.D., 1948-1949
Samuel J. Fogelson, M.D., 1950-1951
Norman G. Parry, M.D., 1952-1953
H. Ivan Sippy, M.D., 1954-1955
Arthur E. Mahle, M.D., 1956-1957
Joseph F. Mallach, M.D., 1958-1959
Edward M. Dorr, M.D., 1960-1961
Durand Smith, M.D., 1962-1963
Clinton L. Compere, M.D., 1964-1965
James B. Hurd, M.D., 1966-1967
Daniel Ruge, M.D., 1968-1969
Melvyn A. Bayly, M.D., 1970-1971
Jacques M. Smith, M.D., 1971-1972

Bibliography

PUBLISHED SOURCES, PROLOGUE

Behan, R.J., M.D., "Development of the Modern Hospital," *Bulletin, American College of Surgeons*, Vol. 24, 1944

Danforth, Isaac Newton, A.M., M.D., *The Life of Nathan Smith Davis, A.M., M.D., LL.D., 1817-1904*, Cleveland Press, 1907 .

Danforth, David Newton, M.D., ed., "Historical Highlights," *Textbook of Obstetrics and Gynecology,* third edition, Harper & Row

Elliott, James Sands, *Outlines of Greek and Roman Medicine,* John Bale, Sons & Danielsson, Ltd., London, 1914

Garrison, Fielding H., *Contributions to the History of Medicine,* Hafner Publishing Co., Philadelphia, 1966

Holmes, Oliver Wendell, "Puerperal Fever as a Private Pestilence," essay published at Harvard University, 1855

Ives, A.G.L., *British Hospitals,* printed in Britain by Clarke & Sherwell LTD Northampton, 1953

Larrabee, Eric, *The Benevolent and Necessary Institution, The New York Hospital, 1771-1971,* Doubleday & Company, Inc. Garden City, New York, 1971

Ludovici, Laurance James, *The Discovery of Anesthesia,* Thomas Y. Crowell Company, New York, 1961

MacEachern, Malcolm T., M.D., F.A.C.H.A., "History of Hospitals," *Hospital Organization and Management,* 1947, second edition

Meyer, Lucy Rider, *Deaconesses,* "Biblical, Early Church, European, American" The Message Publishing Company, Chicago, 1893

Nightingale, Florence, *Notes on Hospitals,* Longman, Roberts and Green, London 1863

Williams, William H., *America's First Hospital: The Pennsylvania Hospital, 1751-1841,* Haverford House, Wayne, Pennsylvania, 1975

Wilson, Grove, *Great Men of Science,* Garden City Publishing Company, 1929

PUBLISHED SOURCES, CHAPTERS 1-27

American Hospital Association, "A Half Century in Retrospect," *Hospitals,* Vol. 22, September, 1948

American Medical Association, "Does Medical Education Need to be Revolutionalized?", *Journal of the AMA,* 19 November 1943

American Medical Association, "Malcolm T. MacEachern," *Journal of the AMA,* 7 April 1962

Arey, Leslie B., *Northwestern University Medical School 1859-1959,* Evanston and Chicago, 1959

Bonner, Thomas Neville, *Medicine in Chicago, 1850-1950,* "Social and Scientific Development of a City," American History Research Center, Madison, Wisconsin, 1957.

Brown, Ray E., "Graduate Education for Hospital Administration," *Foundations and Their Roles*

Brown, Vernon K., *The Story of Passavant Memorial Hospital, 1865-1972,* Chicago, 1977

Bundesen, Herman N., M.D., "One Hundred Years of Public Health," *Illinois Medical Journal,* May, 1940

Cooper, John A.D., M.D., Ph.D., "Undergraduate Medical Education," *Advances in American Medicine,* Josiah Macy Foundation, Jr., for the Bicentennial, 1976

Chicago Hospital Council, "Wesley Memorial Hospital," *Bulletin,* October, 1941

Danforth, David Newton, M.D., "Great Names in Chicago Medicine: Isaac Newton Danforth, M.D.," *Chicago Medicine,* 7 April 1962

Danforth, Isaac N., "Disease Germs," *Chicago Medical Journal,* March, 1872 *William Deering, 1826-1913,* "Historical Sketch" privately printed in Chicago, 1914

Erens, Patricia, *Famous Chicagoans and their Paintings,* "Vizcaya," Chicago Review Press, 1979

Flexner, Abraham, *Medical Education in the United States and Canada,"* Report to the Carnegie Foundation for the Advancement of Teaching," D.B. Updyke, Merrymount Press, Boston, 1910

"E.S. Gilmore, Chicago Hospital Leader," *Modern Hospital*, Vol. 37, 1931

Horton, Isabelle, *High Adventure, Life of Lucy Rider Meyer*, Methodist Book Concern, Cincinnati, 1928

Horton, Isabelle, *The Builders*, The Deaconess Advocate Co., Chicago, 1911

King, William H., *History of Homeopathy and its Institutions in America*, Chicago, 1903

Lewis, Lloyd, and Henry J. Smith, *Chicago: The History of its Reputation*, New York, 1929

Maher, James T., *The Twilight of Splendor, Chronicles of the Age of American Palaces,* "Vizcaya," Little, Brown & Company, Boston and Toronto, 1975

Norton, William Bernard, Ph.D., *The Founding of the Chicago Training School for City, Home and Foreign Missions*, Methodist Historical Society, James Watson & Co., Chicago

Pennewill, Almer M., *The Methodist Movement in Northern Illinois*, 1903

Swift, Louis F., with Arthur Van Vlissingen, *The Yankee of the Yards*, biography of Gustavus Franklin Swift, A.W. Shaw Co., Chicago and New York, 1927

Smith, David S., "Homeopathy in Chicago 1838 to 1865," *Medical Visitor,* January, 1886

Vizcaya, "Guide to the Palace and Gardens," Dade County Art Museum, Miami, Florida, 1977

PUBLISHED SOURCES—CHICAGO WESLEY MEMORIAL HOSPITAL

Annual Reports of Wesley Hospital: 1891, 1892, 1902 through 1913

Annual Reports of Wesley Memorial Hospital: 1914 through 1955

Annual Reports of Chicago Wesley Memorial Hospital: 1956 through 1972

Wesley Memorial Hospital News: a monthly publication from December, 1940 through December, 1943

Wesley Commentator: a news bulletin, December 1944 through 1945

Wesley MEMO: Published every other month for personnel, 1948 through 1972

Wesley Life: published quarterly, 1949 through 1972

NEWSPAPERS

Scrapbooks maintained by the Wesley Woman's Auxiliary 1920-1972 contained numerous news and features about Wesley
  Chicago Daily News
  Chicago Evening Journal
  Chicago Evening Post
  Chicago Today
  Chicago Tribune
  Chicago's American

UPPUBLISHED SOURCES

Charter, 27 October 1888, Constitution and Bylaws of Wesley Hospital

Correspondence: 49 letters from William Deering and James Deering to Wesley Board members, 1905-1923, and replies from Perley Lowe; Letter from Northwestern President William F. McDowell to Wesley Board, 22 September 1914.

Letter from Henry S. Pritchett, President of The Carnegie Foundation, to Perley Lowe, President of Wesley, and Abram W. Harris, President of Northwestern, 11 January 1915

Deed of Land Conveyance from Northwestern University to Wesley Hospital 30 June 1899

Deed of Gift of $1,000,000 from James Deering to Wesley Hospital 9 April 1914

Brief and Argument for Appellees, Wesley Memorial Hospital and James Deering vs. Northwestern University, Appeal in Chancery, Supreme Court of Illinois February 1919

Minutes of the Board of Trustees, Chicago Wesley Memorial Hospital 1960-1972

Minutes of the Ladies Aid Society of Wesley Hospital 1888-1919

Origin and Early Years of Wesley Hospital by Isaac Newton Danforth, 1909

"Fruit of Their Years," a history of the Wesley Woman's Auxiliary from March 20, 1889 through May 31, 1957 by Mrs. Bert J. (May S.) Wilson

Index